Raja Yoga & Yogic Breathing: Two Volume Set

By: William Walker Atkinson

©2021 JD Atlas Books
Cover Photo Credit: Wesley Tingey
Originally Published 1906
For more classic books, visit:
www.jdatlasbooks.com

Introduction

Included in this book bundle are two classics of yoga by prolific author William Walker Atkinson. Mr. Atkinson wrote over one hundred books, ranging from psychology, business, mind reading, yoga, breathing, meditation and more. He also used several pen names depending on the topic of the book. In these two books, *A Series of Lessons in Raja Yoga* and *The Hindu-Yogi Science of Breath*, his pen name was Yogi Ramacharaka.

William originally studied to become an attorney, but due to the stress of the job, he became ill. This illness led to him discovering alternative healing, which he later attributed to the restoration of his health. He became so intrigued, he began writing for a magazine, New Thought.

In the 1890's, Atkinson started studying Hinduism and yoga, which led him to meet and study with popular gurus of his time. This was the time that he wrote the two books included in this bundle.

Raja yoga encompasses both the body and mind, but the emphasis is on mental and spiritual development. The goal is to unite the practitioner with the higher self (enlightenment). Breath is a big component to controlling the mind.

These two books seem to fit perfectly together and we felt readers would appreciate being able to read and reference both together. We sincerely hope you enjoy these two classics.

A Series of Lessons in Raja Yoga

By: William Walker Atkinson

Contents

1 – The "I"

2 – The Ego's Mental Tools

3 – The Expansion of the Self

4 – Mental Control

5 – The Cultivation of Attention

6 – Cultivation of Perception

7 – The Unfoldment of Consciousness

8 – The Highlands and Lowlands of Mind

9 – The Mental Planes

10 – Sub-Consciousing

11 – Sub-Conscious Character Building

12 – Sub-Conscious Influences

THE FIRST LESSON

THE "I."

In India, the Candidates for Initiation into the science of "Raja Yoga," when they apply to the Yogi Masters for instruction, are given a series of lessons designed to enlighten them regarding the nature of the Real Self, and to instruct them in the secret knowledge whereby they may develop the consciousness and realization of the real "I" within them. They are shown how they may cast aside the erroneous or imperfect knowledge regarding their real identity.

Until the Candidate masters this instruction, or at least until the truth becomes fixed in his consciousness, further instruction is denied him, for it is held that until he has awakened to a conscious realization of his Actual Identity, he is not able to understand the source of his power, and, moreover, is not able to *feel* within him the power of the Will, which power underlies the entire teachings of "Raja Yoga."

The Yogi Masters are hot satisfied if the Candidate forms merely a clear intellectual conception of this Actual Identity, but they insist that he must *feel* the truth of the same—must become *aware* of the Real Self—must enter into a consciousness in which the realization becomes a part of his everyday self—in which the realizing consciousness becomes the prevailing idea in his mind, around which his entire thoughts and actions revolve.

To some Candidates, this realization comes like a lightning flash the moment the attention is directed toward it, while in other cases the Candidates find it necessary to follow a rigorous course of training before they acquire the realization in consciousness.

The Yogi Masters teach that there are two degrees of this awakening consciousness of the Real Self. The first, which they call "the Consciousness of the 'I'," is the full consciousness of *real* existence that comes to the Candidate, and which causes him to *know* that he is a real entity having a life not depending upon the body—life that will go on in spite of the destruction of the body—*real* life, in fact. The second degree, which they call "the Consciousness of the 'I AM'," is the consciousness of one's identity with the Universal Life, and his relationship to, and "in-touchness" with all life, expressed and unexpressed. These two degrees of consciousness come in time to all who seek "The Path." To some it comes suddenly; to others it dawns gradually; to many it comes assisted by the exercises and practical work of "Raja Yoga."

The first lesson of the Yogi Masters to the Candidates, leading up to the first degree, above mentioned, is as follows: That the Supreme Intelligence of the Universe—the Absolute—has manifested the being that we call Man—the highest manifestation on this planet. The Absolute has manifested an infinitude of forms of life in the Universe, including distant worlds, suns, planets, etc., many of these forms being unknown to us on this planet, and being impossible of conception by the mind of the ordinary man.

But these lessons have nothing to do with that part of the philosophy which deals with these myriad forms of life, for our time will be taken up with the unfoldment in the mind of man of his true nature and power. Before man attempts to solve the secrets of the Universe without, he should master the Universe within—the Kingdom of the Self. When he has accomplished this, then he may, and should, go forth to gain the outer knowledge as a Master demanding its secrets, rather than as a slave begging for the crumbs from the table of knowledge. The first knowledge for the Candidate is the knowledge of the Self.

Man, the highest manifestation of the Absolute, as far as this planet is concerned, is a wonderfully organized being—although the average man understands but little of his real nature. He comprises within his physical, mental and spiritual make-up both the highest and the lowest, as we have shown in our previous lessons (the "Fourteen Lessons" and the "Advanced Course"). In his bones he manifests almost in the form of mineral life, in fact, in his bones, body and blood mineral substances actually exist. The physical life of the body resembles the life of the plant.

Many of the physical desires and emotions are akin to those of the lower animals, and in the undeveloped man these desires and emotions predominate and overpower the higher nature, which latter is scarcely in evidence. Then Man has a set of mental characteristics that are his own, and which are not possessed by the lower animals (See "Fourteen Lessons").

And in addition to the mental faculties common to all men, or rather, that are in evidence in a greater or lesser degree among all men, there are still higher faculties latent within Man, which when manifested and expressed render Man more than ordinary Man. The unfoldment of these latent faculties is possible to all who have reached the proper stage of development, and the desire and hunger of the student for this instruction is caused by the pressure of these unfolding latent faculties, crying to be born into consciousness. Then there is that wonderful thing, the Will, which is but faintly understood by those ignorant of the Yogi Philosophy—the Power of the Ego—its birthright from the Absolute.

But while these mental and physical things *belong* to Man, they are *not* the Man himself. Before the Man is able to master, control, and direct the things belonging to him—his tools and instruments—he must awaken to a realization of Himself. He must be able to distinguish between the "I" and the "Not I." And this is the first task before the Candidate.

That which is the Real Self of Man is the Divine Spark sent forth from the Sacred Flame. It is the Child of the Divine Parent. It is Immortal—Eternal—Indestructible—Invincible. It possesses within itself Power, Wisdom, and Reality. But like the infant that contains within itself the sometime Man, the mind of Man is unaware of its latent and potential qualities, and does not know itself. As it awakens and unfolds into the knowledge of its real nature, it manifests its qualities, and realizes what the Absolute has given it. When the Real Self begins to awaken, it sets aside from itself those things which are but appendages to it, but which it, in its half-waking state, had regarded as its Self. Setting aside first this, and then that, it finally discards all of the "Not I," leaving the Real Self free and delivered from its bondage to its appendages. Then it returns to the discarded appendages, and makes use of them.

In considering the question: "What is the Real Self?" let us first stop to examine what man usually means when he says "I."

The lower animals do not possess this "I" sense. They are conscious of the outer world; of their own desires and animal cravings and feelings. But their consciousness has not reached the Self-conscious stage. They are not able to think of themselves as separate entities, and to reflect upon their thoughts. They are not possessed of a consciousness of the Divine Spark—the Ego—the Real Self. The Divine Spark is hidden in the lower forms of life—even in the lower forms of human life—by many sheaths that shut out its light. But, nevertheless, it is there, always. It sleeps within the mind of the savage—then, as he unfolds, it begins to throw out its light. In you, the Candidate, it is fighting hard to have its beams pierce through the material coverings When the Real Self begins to arouse itself from its sleep, its dreams vanish from it, and it begins to see the world as it is, and to recognize itself in Reality and not as the distorted thing of its dreams.

The savage and barbarian are scarcely conscious of the "I." They are but a little above the animal in point of consciousness, and their "I" is almost entirely a matter of the consciousness of the wants of the body; the satisfaction of the appetites; the gratification of the passions; the securing of personal comfort; the expression of lust, savage power, etc. In the savage the lower part of the Instinctive Mind is the seat of the "I." (See "Fourteen Lessons" for explanation of the several mental planes of man.) If the savage could analyze his thoughts, he would say that the "I" was the physical body, the said body having certain "feelings," "wants" and "desires." The "I" of such a man is a physical "I," the body representing its form and substance. Not only is this true of the savage, but even among so-called "civilized" men of to-day we find many in this stage. They have developed powers of thinking and reasoning, but they do not "live in their minds" as do some of their brothers. They use their thinking powers for the gratification of their bodily desires and cravings, and really live on the plane of the Instinctive Mind. Such a person may speak of "my mind," or "my soul," not from a high position where he looks upon these things from the standpoint of a Master who realizes his Real Self, but from below, from the point-of-view of the man who lives on the plane of the Instinctive Mind and who sees above *himself* the higher attributes. To such people the body is the "I."

Their "I" is bound up with the senses, and that which comes to them through the senses. Of course, as Man advances in "culture" and "civilization," his senses become educated, and are satisfied only with more refined things, while the less cultivated man is perfectly satisfied with the more material and gross sense gratifications. Much that we call "cultivation" and "culture" is naught but a cultivation of a more refined form of sense gratification, instead of a real advance in consciousness and unfoldment. It is true that the advanced student and Master is possessed of highly developed senses, often far surpassing those of the ordinary man, but in such cases the senses have been cultivated under the mastery of the Will, and are made servants of the Ego instead of things hindering the progress of the soul—they are made servants instead of masters.

As Man advances in the scale, he begins to have a somewhat higher conception of the "I." He begins to use his mind and reason, and he passes on to the Mental Plane—his mind begins to manifest upon the plane of Intellect. He finds that there is something within him that is higher than the body. He finds that his mind seems more *real* to him than does the physical part of him, and in times of deep thought and study he is able almost to forget the existence of the body.

In this second stage, Man soon becomes perplexed. He finds problems that demand an answer, but as soon as he thinks he has answered them the problems present themselves in a new phase, and he is called upon to "explain his explanation." The mind, even although not controlled and directed by the Will, has a wonderful range, but, nevertheless, Man finds himself traveling around and around in a circle, and realizes that he is confronted continually by the Unknown. This disturbs him, and the higher the stage of "book learning" he attains, the more disturbed does he become. The man of but little knowledge does not see the existence of many problems that force themselves before the attention of the man of more knowledge, and demand an explanation from him. The tortures of the man who has attained the mental growth that enables him to see the new problems and the impossibility of their answer, cannot be imagined by one who has not advanced to that stage.

The man in this stage of consciousness thinks of his "I" as a mental thing, having a lower companion, the body. He feels that he has advanced, but yet his "I" does not give him the answer to the riddles and questions that perplex him. And he becomes most unhappy. Such men often develop into Pessimists, and consider the whole of life as utterly evil and disappointing—a curse rather than a blessing. Pessimism belongs to this plane, for neither the Physical Plane man or the Spiritual Plane man have this curse of Pessimism.

The former man has no such disquieting thoughts, for he is almost entirely absorbed in gratifying his animal nature, while the latter man recognizes his mind as an instrument of himself, rather than as *himself*, and knows it to be imperfect in its present stage of growth. He knows that he has in himself the key to all knowledge—locked up in the Ego—and which the trained mind, cultivated, developed and guided by the awakened Will, may grasp as it unfolds. Knowing this the advanced man no longer despairs, and, recognizing his real nature, and his possibilities, as he awakens into a consciousness of his powers and capabilities, he laughs at the old despondent, pessimistic ideas, and discards them like a worn-out garment. Man on the Mental Plane of consciousness is like a huge elephant who knows not his own strength. He could break down barriers and assert himself over nearly any condition or environment, but in his ignorance of his real condition and power he may be mastered by a puny driver, or frightened by the rustling of a piece of paper.

When the Candidate becomes an Initiate—when he passes from the purely Mental Plane on to the Spiritual Plane—he realizes that the "I," the Real Self—is something higher than either body or mind, and that both of the latter may be used as tools and instruments by the Ego or "I." This knowledge is not reached by purely intellectual reasoning, although such efforts of the mind are often necessary to help in the unfoldment, and the Masters so use it. The real knowledge, however, comes as a special form of consciousness. The Candidate becomes "aware" of the real "I," and this consciousness being attained, he passes to the rank of the Initiates. When the Initiate passes the second degree of consciousness, and begins to grow into a realization of his relationship to the Whole—when he begins to manifest the Expansion of Self—then is he on the road to Mastership.

In the present lesson we shall endeavor to point out to the Candidate the methods of developing or increasing the realization of this "I" consciousness—this first-degree work. We give the following exercises or development drills for the Candidate to practice. He will find that a careful and conscientious following of these directions will tend to unfold in him a sufficient degree of the "I" consciousness, to enable him to enter into higher stages of development and power. All that is necessary is for the Candidate to feel within himself the dawn of the awakening consciousness, or awareness of the Real Self. The higher stages of the "I" consciousness come gradually, for once on the Path there is no retrogression or going backward. There may be pauses on the journey, but there is no such thing as actually losing that which is once gained on The Path.

This "I" consciousness, even in its highest stages, is but a preliminary step toward what is called "Illumination," and which signifies the awakening of the Initiate to a realization of his actual connection with and relation to the Whole. The full sight of the glory of the "I," is but a faint reflected glow of "Illumination." The Candidate, once that he enters fully into the "I" consciousness, becomes an "Initiate." And the Initiate who enters into the dawn of Illumination takes his first step upon the road to Mastery.

The Initiation is the awakening of the soul to a knowledge of its real existence — the Illumination is the revelation of the real nature of the soul, and of its relationship with the Whole. After the first dawn of the "I" consciousness has been attained, the Candidate is more able to grasp the means of developing the consciousness to a still higher degree—is more able to use the powers latent within him; to control his own mental states; to manifest a Centre of Consciousness and Influence that will radiate into the outer world which is always striving and hunting for such centers around which it may revolve.

Man must master himself before he can hope to exert an influence beyond himself. There is no royal road to unfoldment and power—each step must be taken in turn, and each Candidate must take the step himself, and by his own effort. But he may, and will, be aided by the helping hand of the teachers who have traveled The Path before him, and who know just when that helping hand is needed to lift the Candidate over the rough places.

We bid the Candidate to pay strict attention to the following instruction, as it is all important. Do not slight any part of it, for we are giving you only what is necessary, and are stating it as briefly as possible. Pay attention, and follow the instruction closely. This lesson must be mastered before you progress. And it must be practiced not only now, but at many stages of the journey, until full Initiation and Illumination is yours.

RULES AND EXERCISES DESIGNED TO AID THE CANDIDATE IN HIS INITIATION

The first instruction along the line of Initiation is designed to awaken the mind to a full realization and consciousness of the individuality of the "I." The Candidate is taught to relax his body, and to calm his mind and to meditate upon the "I" until it is presented clearly and sharply before the consciousness. We herewith give directions for producing the desired physical and mental condition, in which meditation and concentration are more readily practiced. This state of Meditation will be referred to in subsequent exercises, so the Candidate is advised to acquaint himself thoroughly with it.

STATE OF MEDITATION. If possible, retire to a quiet place or room, where you do not fear interruption, so that your mind may feel secure and at rest. Of course, the ideal condition cannot always be obtained, in which case you must do the best you can. The idea is that you should be able to abstract yourself, so far as is possible, from distracting impressions, and you should be alone with yourself—in communion with your Real Self.

It is well to place yourself in an easy chair, or on a couch, so that you may relax the muscles and free the tension of your nerves. You should be able to "let go" all over, allowing every muscle to become limp, until a feeling of perfect peace and restful calm permeates every particle of your being. Rest the body and calm the mind. This condition is best in the earlier stages of the practice, although after the Candidate has acquired a degree of mastery, he will be able to obtain the physical relaxation and mental calm whenever and wherever he desires.

But he must guard against acquiring a "dreamy" way of going around, wrapped in meditation when he should be attending to the affairs of life. *Remember this*, the State of Meditation should be entirely under the control of the Will, and should be entered into only deliberately and at the proper times. The Will must be master of this, as well as of every other mental state. The Initiates are not "day dreamers," but men and women having full control of themselves and their moods. The "I" consciousness while developed by meditation and consciousness, soon becomes a fixed item of consciousness, and does not have to be produced by meditation. In time of trial, doubt, or trouble, the consciousness may be brightened by an effort of the Will (as we shall explain in subsequent lessons) without going into the State of Meditation.

THE REALIZATION OF THE "I." The Candidate must first acquaint himself with the reality of the "I," before he will be able to learn its real nature. This is the first step. Let the Candidate place himself in the State of Meditation, as heretofore described.

Then let him concentrate his entire attention upon his Individual Self, shutting out all thought of the outside world, and other persons. Let him form in his mind the idea of himself as a *real* thing—an actual being—an individual entity—a Sun around which revolves the world. He must see himself as the Centre around which the whole world revolves. Let not a false modesty, or sense of depreciation interfere with this idea, for you are not denying the right of others to also consider themselves centers. You are, in fact, a center of consciousness—made so by the Absolute—and you are awakening to the fact. Until the Ego recognizes itself as a Centre of Thought, Influence and Power, it will not be able to *manifest* these qualities. And in proportion as it recognizes its position as a center, so will it be able to manifest its qualities. It is not necessary that you should compare yourself with others, or imagine yourself greater or higher than them.

In fact, such comparisons are to be regretted, and are unworthy of the advanced Ego, being a mark and indication of a lack of development, rather than the reverse. In the Meditation simply ignore all consideration of the respective qualities of others, and endeavor to realize the fact that YOU are a great Centre of Consciousness—a Centre of Power—a Centre of Influence—a Centre of Thought. And that like the planets circling around the sun, so does your world revolve around YOU who are its center. It will not be necessary for you to argue out this matter, or to convince yourself of its truth by intellectual reasoning. The knowledge does not come in that way. It comes in the shape of a realization of the truth gradually dawning upon your consciousness through meditation and concentration. Carry this thought of yourself as a "Centre of Consciousness—Influence—Power" with you, *for it is an occult truth,* and in the proportion that you are able, to realize it so will be your ability to manifest the qualities named.

No matter how humble may be your position—no matter how hard may be your lot—no matter how deficient in educational advantages you may be—still you would not change your "I" with the most fortunate, wisest and highest man or woman in the world. You may doubt this, but think for a moment and you will see that we are right. When you say that you "would like to be" this person or that, you really mean that *you* would like to have their degree of intelligence, power, wealth, position, or what not. What you want is something that is theirs, or something akin to it. But you would not for a moment wish to merge your *identity* with theirs, or to exchange *selves.* Think of this for a moment To *be* the other person you would have to let *yourself* die, and instead of *yourself* you would be the other person. The real *you* would be wiped out of existence, and you would not be *you* at all, but would be *he.*

If you can but grasp this idea you will see that not for a moment would you be willing for such an exchange. Of course, such an exchange is impossible. The "I" of you cannot be wiped out. It is eternal, and will go on, and on, and on, to higher and higher states—but it always will be the same "I." Just as you, although a far different sort of person from your childhood self, still you recognize that the same "I" is there, and always has been there. And although you will attain knowledge, experience, power and wisdom in the coming years, the same "I" will be there. The "I" is the Divine Spark and cannot be extinguished.

The majority of people in the present stage of the race development have but a faint conception of the reality of the "I." They accept the statement of its existence, and are conscious of themselves as an eating, sleeping, living creature—something like a higher form of animal. But they have not awakened to an "awareness" or realization of the "I," which must come to all who become real centers of Influence and Power. Some men have stumbled into this consciousness, or a degree of it, without understanding the matter. They have "felt" the truth of it, and they have stepped out from the ranks of the commonplace people of the world, and have become powers for good or bad. This is unfortunate to some extent, as this "awareness" without the knowledge that should accompany it may bring pain to the individual and others.

The Candidate must meditate upon the "I," and recognize it—*feel* it—to be a Centre. This is his first task. Impress upon your mind the word "I," in this sense and understanding, and let it sink deep down into your consciousness, so that it will become a part of you. And when you say "I," you must accompany the word with the picture of your Ego as a Centre of Consciousness, and Thought, and Power, and Influence. See yourself thus, surrounded by your world. Wherever you go, there goes the Centre of your world. YOU are the Centre, and all outside of you revolves around that Centre. This is the first great lesson on the road to Initiation. Learn it!

The Yogi Masters teach the Candidates that their realization of the "I" as a Centre may be hastened by going into the Silence, or State of Meditation, and repeating their first name over slowly, deliberately and solemnly a number of times. This exercise tends to cause the mind to center upon the "I," and many cases of dawning Initiation have resulted from this practice. Many original thinkers have stumbled upon this method, without having been taught it. A noted example is that of Lord Tennyson, who has written that he attained a degree of Initiation in this way. He would repeat his own name, over and over, and the same time meditating upon his identity, and he reports that he would become conscious and "aware" of his reality and immortality—in short would recognize himself as a *real* center of consciousness.

We think we have given you the key to the first stage of meditation and concentration. Before passing on, let us quote from one of the old Hindu Masters. He says, regarding this matter: "When the soul sees itself as a Centre surrounded by its circumference—when the Sun knows that it is a Sun, and is surrounded by its whirling planets—then is it ready for the Wisdom and Power of the Masters."

THE KNOWLEDGE OF THE INDEPENDENCE OF THE "I" FROM THE BODY

Many of the Candidates find themselves prevented from a full realization of the "I" (even after they have begun to grasp it) by the confusing of the reality of the "I" with the sense of the physical body. This is a stumbling block that is easily overcome by meditation and concentration, the independence of the "I" often becoming manifest to the Candidate in a flash, upon the proper thought being used as the subject of meditation.

The exercise is given as follows: Place yourself in the State of Meditation, and think of YOURSELF—the Real "I"—as being independent of the body, but using the body as a covering and an instrument. Think of the body as you might of a suit of clothes. Realize that you are able to leave the body, and still be the same "I." Picture yourself as doing this, and looking down upon your body. Think of the body as a shell from which you may emerge without affecting your identity. Think of yourself as mastering and controlling the body that you occupy, and using it to the best advantage, making it healthy, strong and vigorous, but still being merely a shell or covering for the real "You." Think of the body as composed of atoms and cells which are constantly changing, but which are held together by the force of your Ego, and which you can improve at Will. Realize that you are merely inhabiting the body, and using it for your convenience, just as you might use a house.

In meditating further, ignore the body entirely, and place your thought upon the Real "I" that you are beginning to feel to be "you," and you will find that your identity—your "I"—is something entirely apart from the body. You may now say "my body" with a new meaning. Divorce the idea of your being a physical being, and realize that you are above body. But do not let this conception and realization cause you to ignore the body. You must regard the body as the Temple of the Spirit, and care for it, and make it a fit habitation for the "I." Do not be frightened if, during this meditation, you happen to experience the sensation of being out of the body for a few moments, and of returning to it when you are through with the exercise. The Ego is able (in the case of the advanced Initiate) of soaring above the confines of the body, but it never severs its connection at such times. It is merely as if one were to look out of the window of a room, seeing what was going on outside, and drawing in his head when he wishes. He does not leave the room, although he may place his head outside in order to observe what is doing in the street. We do not advise the Candidate to try to cultivate this sensation—but if it comes naturally during meditation, do not fear.

REALIZING THE IMMORTALITY AND INVINCIBILITY OF THE EGO

While the majority accept on faith the belief in the Immortality of the Soul, yet but few are aware that it may be demonstrated by the soul itself. The Yogi Masters teach the Candidates this lesson, as follows: The Candidate places himself in the State of Meditation, or at least in a thoughtful frame of mind, and then endeavors to "imagine" himself as "dead"—that is, he tries to form a mental conception of himself as dead. This, at first thought, appears a very easy thing to imagine, but as a matter of fact it is *impossible* to do so, for the Ego refuses to entertain the proposition, and finds it impossible to imagine it. Try it for yourself. You will find that you may be able to imagine your *body* as lying still and lifeless, but the same thought finds that in so doing *You* are standing and looking at the body. So you see that *You* are not dead at all, even in imagination, although the body may be. Or, if you refuse to disentangle yourself from your body, in imagination, you may think of your body as dead but *You* who refuse to leave it are still *alive* and recognize the dead body as a thing apart from your Real Self.

No matter how you may twist it you *cannot* imagine yourself as dead. The Ego insists upon being *alive* in any of these thoughts, and thus finds that it has within itself the sense and assurance of Immortality. In case of sleep or stupor resulting from a blow, or from narcotics or anesthetics, the mind is apparently blank, but the "I" is conscious of a continuity of existence. And so, one may imagine himself as being in an unconscious state, or asleep, quite easily, and sees the possibility of such a state, but when it comes to imagining the "I" as dead, the mind utterly refuses to do the work. This wonderful fact that the soul carries within itself the evidence of its own immortality is a glorious thing, but one must have reached a degree of unfoldment before he is able to grasp its full significance.

The Candidate is advised to investigate the above statement for himself, by meditation and concentration, for in order that the "I" may know its true nature and possibilities, it must realize that it cannot be destroyed or killed. It must know what it is before it is able to manifest its nature. So do not leave this part of the teaching until you have mastered it. And it is well occasionally to return to it, in order that you may impress upon the mind the fact of your immortal and eternal nature. The mere glimmering of this conception of truth will give you an increased sense of strength and power, and you will find that your Self has expanded and grown, and that you are more of a power and Centre than you have heretofore realized.

The following exercises are useful in bringing about a realization of the invincibility of the Ego—its superiority to the elements.

Place yourself in the State of Meditation, and imagine the "I" as withdrawn from the body. See it passing through the tests of air, fire and water unharmed. The body being out of the way, the soul is seen to be able of passing through the air at will—of floating like a bird—of soaring—of traveling in the ether. It may be seen as able to pass through fire without harm and without sensation, for the elements affect only the physical body, not the Real "I." Likewise it may be seen as passing through water without discomfort or danger or hurt.

This meditation will give you a sense of superiority and strength, and will show you something of the nature of the real "I." It is true that you are confined in the body, and the body may be affected by the elements, but the knowledge that the Real "I" is superior to the body—superior to the elements that affect the body—and cannot be injured any more than it can be killed, is wonderful, and tends to develop the full "I" consciousness within you. For You—the Real "I"—are not body. You are Spirit.

The Ego is Immortal and Invincible, and cannot be killed and harmed. When you enter into this realization and consciousness, you will feel an influx of strength and power impossible to describe. Fear will fall from you like a worn-out cloak, and you will feel that you are "born again." An understanding of this thought, will show you that the things that we have been fearing cannot affect the Real "I," but must rest content with hurting the physical body. And they may be warded off from the physical body by a proper understanding and application of the Will.

In our next lesson, you will be taught how to separate the "I" from the mechanism of the mind—how you may realize your mastery of the mind, just as you now realize your independence of the body. This knowledge must be imparted to you by degrees, and you must place your feet firmly upon one round of the ladder before you take the next step.

The watchword of this First Lesson is "I." And the Candidate must enter fully into its meaning before he is able to progress. He must realize his real existence—independent of the body. He must see himself as invincible and impervious to harm, hurt, or death. He must see himself as a great Centre of Consciousness—a Sun around which his world revolves. Then will come to him a new strength. He will feel a calm dignity and power, which will be apparent to those with whom he comes in contact. He will be able to look the world in the face without flinching, and without fear, for he will realize the nature and power of the "I." He will realize that he is a Centre of Power—of Influence. He will realize that nothing can harm the "I," and that no matter how the storms of life may dash upon the personality, the real "I"—the Individuality—is unharmed. Like a rock that stands steadfast throughout the storm, so does the "I" stand through the tempests of the life of personality. And he will know that as he grows in realization, he will be able to control these storms and bid them be still.

In the words of one of the Yogi Masters: "The 'I' is eternal. It passes unharmed through the fire, the air, the water. Sword and spear cannot kill or wound it. It cannot die. The trials of the physical life are but as dreams to it. Resting secure in the knowledge of the 'I,' Man may smile at the worst the world has to offer, and raising his hand he may bid them disappear into the mist from which they emerged. Blessed is he who can say (understandingly) 'I'."

So dear Candidate, we leave you to master the First Lesson. Be not discouraged if your progress be slow. Be not cast down if you slip back a step after having gained it. You will gain two at the next step. Success and realization will be yours. Mastery is before. You will Attain. You will Accomplish. Peace be with you.

MANTRAMS (AFFIRMATIONS) FOR THE FIRST LESSON

"I" am a Centre. Around me revolves my world.

"I" am a Centre of Influence and Power.

"I" am a Centre of Thought and Consciousness.

"I" am Independent of the Body.

"I" am Immortal and cannot be Destroyed.

"I" am Invincible and cannot be Injured.

THE SECOND LESSON

THE EGO'S MENTAL TOOLS.

In the First Lesson we gave instruction and exercises designed to awaken the consciousness of the Candidate to a realization of the real "I." We confined our instructions to the preliminary teachings of the reality of the "I," and the means whereby the Candidate might be brought to a realization of his real Self, and its independence from the body and the things of the flesh. We tried to show you how you might awaken to a consciousness of the reality of the "I"; its real nature; its independence of the body; its immortality; its invincibility and invulnerability. How well we have succeeded may be determined only by the experience of each Candidate, for we can but point out the way, and the Candidate must do the real work himself.

But there is more to be said and done in this matter of awakening to a realization of the "I." So far, we have but told you how to distinguish between the material coverings of the Ego and the "I" itself. We have tried to show you that you had a real "I," and then to show you what it was, and how it was independent of the material coverings, etc. But there is still another step in this self-analysis—a more difficult step. Even when the Candidate has awakened to a realization of his independence of the body, and material coverings, he often confounds the "I" with the lower principles of the mind. This is a mistake.

The Mind, in its various phases and planes, is but a tool and instrument of the "I," and is far from being the "I" itself. We shall try to bring out this fact in this lesson and its accompanying exercises. We shall avoid, and pass by, the metaphysical features of the case, and shall confine ourselves to the Yogi Psychology. We shall not touch upon theories, nor attempt to explain the cause, nature and purpose of the Mind— the working tool of the Ego—but instead shall attempt to point out a way whereby you may analyze the Mind and then determine which is the "not I" and which is the real "I." It is useless to burden you with theories or metaphysical talk, when the way to prove the thing is right within your own grasp. By using the mind, you will be able to separate it into its parts, and force it to give you its own answer to the questions touching itself.

In the second and third lessons of our *Fourteen Lessons*, we pointed out to you the fact that man had three Mental Principles, or subdivisions of mind, all of which were below the plane of Spirit. The "I" is Spirit, but its mental principles are of a lower order. Without wishing to unduly repeat ourselves, we think it better to run hastily over these three Principles in the mind of Man.

First, there is what is known as the Instinctive Mind, which man shares in common with the lower animals. It is the first principle of mind that appears in the scale of evolution. In its lowest phases, consciousness is but barely perceptible, and mere sensation is apparent. In its higher stages it almost reaches the plane of Reason or Intellect, in fact, they overlap each other, or, rather, blend into each other. The Instinctive Mind does valuable work in the direction of maintaining animal life in our bodies, it having charge of this part of our being. It attends to the constant work of repair; replacement; change; digestion; assimilation; elimination, etc., all of which work is performed below the plane of consciousness.

But this is but a small part of the work of the Instinctive Mind. For this part of the mind has stored up all the experiences of ourselves and ancestors in our evolution from the lower forms of animal life into the present stage of evolution. All of the old animal instincts (which were all right in their place, and quite necessary for the well-being of the lower forms of life) have left traces in this part of the mind, which traces are apt to come to the front under pressure of unusual circumstances, even long after we think we have outgrown them.

In this part of the mind are to be found traces of the old fighting instinct of the animal; all the animal passions; all the hate, envy, jealousy, and the rest of it, which are our inheritances from the past. The Instinctive Mind is also the "habit mind" in which is stored up all the little, and great, habits of many lives, or rather such as have not been entirely effaced by subsequent habits of a stronger nature. The Instinctive Mind is a queer storehouse, containing quite a variety of objects, many of them very good in their way, but others of which are the worst kind of old junk and rubbish.

This part of the mind also is the seat of the appetites; passions; desires; instincts; sensations; feelings and emotions of the lower order, manifested in the lower animals; primitive man; the barbarian; and the man of today, the difference being only in the degree of control over them that has been gained by the higher parts of the mind. There are higher desires, aspirations, etc., belonging to a higher part of the mind, which we will describe in a few minutes, but the "animal nature" belongs to the Instinctive Mind.

To it also belong the "feelings" belonging to our emotional and passional nature. All animal desires, such as hunger and thirst; sexual desires (on the physical plane); all passions, such as physical love; hatred; envy; malice; jealousy; revenge, etc., are part of this part of the mind. The desire for the physical (unless a means of reaching higher things) and the longing for the material, belong to this region of the mind. The "lust of the flesh; the lust of the eyes; the pride of life," belong to the Instinctive Mind.

Take note, however, that we are not condemning the things belonging to this plane of the mind. All of them have their place—many were necessary in the past, and many are still necessary for the continuance of physical life. All are right in their place, and to those in the particular plane of development to which they belong, and are wrong only when one is mastered by them, or when he returns to pick up an unworthy thing that has been cast off in the unfoldment of the individual. This lesson has nothing to do with the right and wrong of these things (we have treated of that elsewhere) and we mention this part of the mind that you may understand that you have such a thing in your mental make-up, and that you may understand the thought, etc., coming from it, when we start in to analyze the mind in the latter part of this lesson. All we will ask you to do at this stage of the lesson is to realize that this part of the mind, while *belonging* to you, is *not* You, yourself. It is *not* the "I" part of you.

Next in order, above the Instinctive Mind, is what we have called the Intellect, that part of the mind that does our reasoning, analyzing; "thinking," etc. You are using it in the consideration of this lesson. But note this: You are *using* it, but it is *not* You, any more than was the Instinctive Mind that you considered a moment ago. You will begin to make the separation, if you will think but a moment. We will not take up your time with a consideration of Intellect or Reason. You will find a good description of this part of the mind in any good elementary work on Psychology. Our only idea in mentioning it is that you may make the classification, and that we may afterward show you that the Intellect is but a tool of the Ego, instead of being the real "I" itself, as so many seem to imagine.

The third, and highest, Mental Principle is what is called the Spiritual Mind, that part of the mind which is almost unknown to many of the race, but which has developed into consciousness with nearly all who read this lesson, for the fact that the subject of this lesson attracts you is a proof that this part of your mental nature is unfolding into consciousness. This region of the mind is the source of that which we call "genius," "inspiration," "spirituality," and all that we consider the "highest" in our mental make-up.

All the great thoughts and ideas float into the field of consciousness from this part of the mind. All the great unfoldment of the race comes from there. All the higher mental ideas that have come to Man in his upward evolutionary journey, that tend in the direction of nobility; true religious feeling; kindness; humanity; justice; unselfish love; mercy; sympathy, etc., have come to him through his slowly unfolding Spiritual Mind. His love of God and of his fellow man have come in this way. His knowledge of the great occult truths reaches him through this channel. The mental realization of the "I," which we are endeavoring to teach in these lessons, must come to him by way of the Spiritual Mind unfolding its ideas into his field of consciousness.

But even this great and wonderful part of the mind is but a tool—a highly finished one, it is true, but still a tool—to the Ego, or "I."

We propose to give you a little mental drill work, toward the end that you may be able more readily to distinguish the "I" from the mind, or mental states. In this connection we would say that every part, plane, and function of the mind is good, and necessary, and the student must not fall into the error of supposing that because we tell him to set aside first this part of the mind and then that part, that we are undervaluing the mind, or that we regard it as an encumbrance or hindrance. Far from this, we realize that it is *by the use of* the mind that Man is enabled to arrive at a knowledge of his true nature and Self, and that his progress through many stages yet will depend upon the unfolding of his mental faculties.

Man is now using but the lower and inferior parts of his mind, and he has within his mental world great unexplored regions that far surpass anything of which the human mind has dreamed. In fact, it is part of the business of "Raja Yoga" to aid in unfolding these higher faculties and mental regions. And so far from decrying the Mind, the "Raja Yoga" teachers are chiefly concerned in recognizing the Mind's power and possibilities, and directing the student to avail himself of the latent powers that are inherent in his soul.

It is only by the mind that the teachings we are now giving you may be grasped and understood, and used to your advantage and benefit. We are talking direct to your mind now, and are making appeals to it, that it may be interested and may open itself to what is ready to come into it from its own higher regions. We are appealing to the Intellect to direct its attention to this great matter, that it may interpose less resistance to the truths that are waiting to be projected from the Spiritual Mind, which knows the Truth.

MENTAL DRILL

Place yourself in a calm, restful condition, that you may be able to meditate upon the matters that we shall place before you for consideration. Allow the matters presented to meet with a hospitable reception from you, and hold a mental attitude of willingness to receive what may be waiting for you in the higher regions of your mind.

We wish to call your attention to several mental impressions or conditions, one after another, in order that you may realize that they are merely something *incident* to you, and *not* YOU yourself—that you may set them aside and consider them, just as you might anything that you have been using. You cannot set the "I" aside and so consider it, but the various forms of the "not I" may be so set aside and considered.

In the First Lesson you gained the perception of the "I" as independent from the body, the latter merely being an instrument for use. You have now arrived at the stage when the "I" appears to you to be a mental creature—a bundle of thoughts, feelings, moods, etc. But you must go farther. You must be able to distinguish the "I" from these mental conditions, which are as much tools as is the body and its parts.

Let us begin by considering the thoughts more closely connected with the body, and then work up to the higher mental states.

The sensations of the body, such as hunger; thirst; pain; pleasurable sensations; physical desires, etc., etc., are not apt to be mistaken for essential qualities of the "I" by many of the Candidates, for they have passed beyond this stage, and have learned to set aside these sensations, to a greater or lesser extent, by an effort of the Will, and are no longer slaves to them. Not that they do not experience these sensations, but they have grown to regard them as incidents of the physical life—good in their place—but useful to the advanced man only when he has mastered them to the extent that he no longer regards them as close to the "I."

And yet, to some people, these sensations are so closely identified with their conception of the "I" that when they think of themselves, they think merely of a bundle of these sensations. They are not able to set them aside and consider them as things apart, to be used when necessary and proper, but as things not fastened to the "I." The more advanced a man becomes the farther off seem these sensations. Not that he does not feel hungry, for instance. Not at all, for he recognizes hunger, and satisfies it within reason, knowing that his physical body is making demands for attention, and that these demands should be heeded.

But—mark the difference—instead of feeling that the "*I*" is hungry the man feels that "*my body*" is hungry, just as he might become conscious that his horse or dog was crying for food insistently. Do you see what we mean? It is that the man no longer identifies himself—the "I"—with the body, consequently the thoughts which are most closely allied to the physical life seem comparatively "separate" from his "I" conception. Such a man thinks "my stomach, this," or "my leg, that," or "my body, thus," instead of "'I,' this," or "'I' that." He is able, almost automatically, to think of the body and its sensations as things *of* him, and *belonging to* him, which require attention and care, rather than as real parts of the "I." He is able to form a conception of the "I" as existing without any of these things—without the body and its sensations—and so he has taken the first step in the realization of the "I."

Before going on, we ask the students to stop a few moments, and mentally run over these sensations of the body. Form a mental image of them, and realize that they are merely incidents to the present stage of growth and experience of the "I," and that they form no real part of it. They may, and will be, left behind in the Ego's higher planes of advancement. You may have attained this mental conception perfectly, long since, but we ask that to give yourself the mental drill at this time, in order to fasten upon your mind this first step.

In realizing that you are able to set aside, mentally, these sensations—that you are able to hold them out at arm's length and "consider" them as an "outside" thing, you mentally determine that they are "not I" things, and you set them down in the "not I" collection—the first to be placed there. Let us try to make this still plainer, even at the risk of wearying you by repetitions (for you must get this idea firmly fixed in your mind). To be able to say that a thing is "not I," you must realize that there are two things in question (1) the "not I" thing, and (2) the "I" who is regarding the "not I" thing just as the "I" regards a lump of sugar, or a mountain. Do you see what we mean? Keep at it until you do.

Next, consider some of the emotions, such as anger; hate; love, in its ordinary forms; jealousy; ambition; and the hundred and one other emotions that sweep through our brains. You will find that you are able to set each one of these emotions or feelings aside and study it; dissect it; analyze it; consider it. You will be able to understand the rise, progress and end of each of these feelings, as they have come to you, and as you recall them in your memory or imagination, just as readily as you would were you observing their occurrence in the mind of a friend. You will find them all stored away in some parts of your mental make-up, and you may (to use a modern American slang phrase) "make them trot before you, and show their paces." Don't you see that they are not "You"—that they are merely something that you carry around with you in a mental bag. You can imagine yourself as living without them, and still being "I," can you not?

And the very fact that you are able to set them aside and examine and consider them is a proof that they are "not I" things—for there are two things in the matter (1) *You* who are examining and considering them, and (2) the thing itself which is the *object* of the examination and consideration at mental arm's length. So into the "not I" collection go these emotions, desirable and undesirable. The collection is steadily growing, and will attain quite formidable proportions after a while.

Now, do not imagine that this is a lesson designed to teach you how to discard these emotions, although if it enables you to get rid of the undesirable ones, so much the better. This is not our object, for we bid you place the desirable (at this time) ones in with the opposite kind, the idea being to bring you to a realization that the "I" is higher, above and independent of these mental somethings, and then when you have realized the nature of the "I," you may return and use (as a Master) the things that have been using you as a slave.

So, do not be afraid to throw these emotions (good and bad) into the "not I" collection. You may go back to them, and use the good ones, after the Mental Drill is over. No matter how much you may think that you are bound by any of these emotions, you will realize, by careful analysis, that it is of the "not I" kind, for the "I" existed before the emotion came into active play, and it will live long after the emotion has faded away. The principal proof is that you are able to hold it out at arm's length and examine it—a proof that it is "not I."

Run through the entire list of your feelings; emotions; moods; and what not, just as you would those of a well-known friend or relative, and you will see that each one—every one—is a "not I" thing, and you will lay it aside for the time, for the purpose of the scientific experiment, at least.

Then passing on to the Intellect, you will be able to hold out for examination each mental process and principle. You don't believe it, you may say. Then read and study some good work on Psychology, and you will learn to dissect and analyze every intellectual process—and to classify it and place it in the proper pigeon-hole. Study Psychology by means of some good text-book, and you will find that one by one every intellectual process is classified, and talked about and labeled, just as you would a collection of flowers.

If that does not satisfy you, turn the leaves of some work on Logic, and you will admit that you may hold these intellectual processes at arm's length and examine them, and talk about them to others. So that these wonderful tools of Man—the Intellectual powers may be placed in the "not I" collection, for the "I" is capable of standing aside and viewing them—it is able to detach them from itself. The most remarkable thing about this is that in admitting this fact, you realize that the "I" is using these very intellectual faculties to pass upon themselves. Who is the Master that compels these faculties to do this to themselves? The Master of the Mind—The "I."

And reaching the higher regions of the mind—even the Spiritual Mind, you will be compelled to admit that the things that have come into consciousness from that region may be considered and studied, just as may be any other mental thing, and so even these high things must be placed in the "not I" collection. You may object that this does not prove that all the things in the Spiritual Mind may be so treated—that there maybe "I" things there that cannot be so treated.

We will not discuss this question, for you know nothing about the Spiritual Mind except as it has revealed itself to you, and the higher regions of that mind are like the mind of a God, when compared to what *you* call mind. But the evidence of the Illumined—those in whom the Spiritual Mind has wonderfully unfolded tell us that even in the highest forms of development, the Initiates, yea, even the Masters, realize that above even their highest mental states there is always that eternal "I" brooding over them, as the Sun over the lake; and that the highest conception of the "I" known even to advanced souls, is but a faint reflection of the "I" filtering through the Spiritual Mind, although that Spiritual Mind is as clear as the clearest crystal when compared with our comparatively opaque mental states. And the highest mental state is but a tool or instrument of the "I," and is not the "I" itself.

And yet the "I" is to be found in the faintest forms of consciousness, and animates even the unconscious life. The "I" is always the same, but its apparent growth is the result of the mental unfoldment of the individual. As we described it in one of the lessons of the "*Advanced Course*" it is like an electric lamp that is encased in many wrappings of cloth. As cloth after cloth is removed, the light seems to grow brighter and stronger, and yet it has changed not, the change being in the removal of the confining and bedimming coverings.

We do not expect to make you realize the "I" in all its fullness—that is far beyond the highest known to man of to-day—but we do hope to bring you to a realization of the highest conception of the "I," possible to each of you in your present stage of unfoldment, and in the process, we expect to cause to drop from you some of the confining sheaths that you have about outgrown. The sheaths are ready for dropping, and all that is required is the touch of a friendly hand to cause them to fall fluttering from you. We wish to bring you to the fullest possible (to you) realization of the "I," in order to make an Individual of you—in order that you may understand, and have courage to take up the tools and instruments lying at your hand, and do the work before you.

And now, back to the Mental Drill. After you have satisfied yourself that about everything that you are capable of thinking about is a "not I" thing—a tool and instrument for your use—you will ask, "And now, what is there left that should not be thrown in the "not I" collection." To this question we answer "THE 'I' ITSELF." And when you demand a proof we say, "Try to set aside the 'I' for consideration!" You may try from now until the passing away of infinities of infinities, and you will never be able to set aside the real "I" for consideration. You may think you can, but a little reflection will show you that you are merely setting aside some of your mental qualities or faculties. And in this process what is the "I" doing? Simply setting aside and considering things. Can you not see that the "I" cannot be both the *considerer* and the thing considered—the *examiner* and the thing examined? Can the sun shine upon itself by its own light?

You may consider the "I" of some other person, but it is *your* "I" that is considering. But you cannot, as an "I," stand aside and see yourself as an "I." Then what evidence have we that there is an "I" to us? This: that you are always conscious of being the considerer and examiner, instead of the considered and examined thing—and then, you have the evidence of your consciousness. And what report does this consciousness give us? Simply this, and nothing more: "I AM." That is all that the "I" is conscious of, regarding its true self: "I AM," but that consciousness is worth all the rest, for the rest is but "not I" tools that the "I" may reach out and use.

And so, at the final analysis, you will find that there is something that refuses to be set aside and examined by the "I." And that something is the "I" itself—that "I" eternal, unchangeable—that drop of the Great Spirit Ocean—that spark from the Sacred Flame.

Just as you find it impossible to imagine the "I" as dead, so will you find it impossible to set aside the "I" for consideration—all that comes to you is the testimony: "I AM."

If you were able to set aside the "I" for consideration, who would be the one to consider it? Who could consider except the "I" itself, and if it be *here*, how could it be *there?* The "I" cannot be the "not I" even in the wildest flights of the imagination—the imagination with all its boasted freedom and power, confesses itself vanquished when asked to do this thing.

Oh, students, may you be brought to a realization of what you are. May you soon awaken to the fact that you are sleeping gods—that you have within you the power of the Universe, awaiting your word to manifest in action. Long ages have you toiled to get this far, and long must you travel before you reach even the first Great Temple, but you are now entering into the conscious stage of Spiritual Evolution. No longer will your eyes be closed as you walk the Path. From now on you will begin to see clearer and clearer each step, in the dawning light of consciousness.

You are in touch with all of life, and the separation of your "I" from the great Universal "I" is but apparent and temporary. We will tell you of these things in our

Third Lesson, but before you can grasp that you must develop the "I" consciousness within you. Do not lay aside this matter as one of no importance. Do not dismiss our weak explanation as being "merely words, words, words," as so many are inclined to do. We are pointing out a great truth to you. Why not follow the leadings of the Spirit which even now—this moment while you read—is urging you to walk The Path of Attainment? Consider the teachings of this lesson, and practice the Mental Drill until your mind has grasped its significance, then let it sink deep down into your inner consciousness. Then will you be ready for the next lessons, and those to follow.

Practice this Mental Drill until you are fully assured of the *reality* of the "I" and the *relativity* of the "not "I" in the mind. When you once grasp this truth, you will find that you will be able to use the mind with far greater power and effect, for you will recognize that it is your tool and instrument, fitted and intended to do your bidding. You will be able to master your moods, and emotions when necessary, and will rise from the position of a slave to a Master.

Our words seem cheap and poor, when we consider the greatness of the truth that we are endeavoring to convey by means of them. For who can find words to express the inexpressible? All that we may hope to do is to awaken a keen interest and attention on your part, so that you will practice the Mental Drill, and thus obtain the evidence of your own mentality to the truth. Truth is not truth to you until you have proven it in your own experience, and once so proven you cannot be robbed of it, nor can it be argued away from you.

You must realize that in every mental effort You—the "I"—are behind it. You bid the Mind work, and it obeys your Will. You are the Master, and not the slave of your mind. You are the Driver, not the driven. Shake yourself loose from the tyranny of the mind that has oppressed you for so long. Assert yourself, and be free. We will help you in this direction during the course of these lessons, but you must first assert yourself as a Master of your Mind. Sign the mental Declaration of Independence from your moods, emotions, and uncontrolled thoughts, and assert your Dominion over them. Enter into your Kingdom, thou manifestation of the Spirit!

While this lesson is intended primarily to bring clearly into your consciousness the fact that the "I" is a reality, separate and distinct from its Mental Tools, and while the control of the mental faculties by the Will forms a part of some of the future lessons, still, we think that this is a good place to point out to you the advantages arising from a realization of the true nature of the "I" and the relative aspect of the Mind.

Many of us have supposed that our minds were the masters of ourselves, and we have allowed ourselves to be tormented and worried by thoughts "running away" with us, and presenting themselves at inopportune moments. The Initiate is relieved from this annoyance, for he learns to assert his mastery over the different parts of the mind, and controls and regulates his mental processes, just as one would a fine piece of machinery. He is able to control his conscious thinking faculties, and direct their work to the best advantage, and he also learns how to pass on orders to the subconscious mental region and bid it work for him while he sleeps, or even when he is using his conscious mind in other matters. These subjects will be considered by us in due time, during the course of lessons.

In this connection it may be interesting to read what Edward Carpenter says of the power of the individual to control his thought processes. In his book "*From Adam's Peak to Eleplumta,*" in describing his experience while visiting a Hindu Gnani Yogi, he says:

"And if we are unwilling to believe in this internal mastery over the body, we are perhaps almost equally unaccustomed to the idea of mastery over our own inner thoughts and feelings. That a man should be a prey to any thought that chances to take possession of his mind, is commonly among us assumed as unavoidable. It may be a matter of regret that he should be kept awake all night from anxiety as to the issue of a lawsuit on the morrow, but that he should have the power of determining whether he be kept awake or not seems an extravagant demand. The image of an impending calamity is no doubt odious, but its very odiousness (we say) makes it haunt the mind all the more pertinaciously and it is useless to try to expel it.

"Yet this is an absurd position—for man, the heir of all the ages: hag-ridden by the flimsy creatures of his own brain. If a pebble in our boot torments us, we expel it. We take off the boot and shake it out. And once the matter is fairly understood it is just as easy to expel an intruding and obnoxious thought from the mind. About this there ought to be no mistake, no two opinions. The thing is obvious, clear and unmistakable. It should be as easy to expel an obnoxious thought from your mind as it is to shake a stone out of your shoe; and till a man can do that it is just nonsense to talk about his ascendancy over Nature, and all the rest of it. He is a mere slave, and prey to the bat-winged phantoms that flit through the corridors of his own brain.

"Yet the weary and careworn faces that we meet by thousands, even among the affluent classes of civilization, testify only too clearly how seldom this mastery is obtained. How rare indeed to meet a *man*! How common rather to discover a creature hounded on by tyrant thoughts (or cares or desires), cowering, wincing under the lash—or perchance priding himself to run merrily in obedience to a driver that rattles the reins and persuades him that he is free—whom we cannot converse with in careless *tete-a-tete* because that alien presence is always there, on the watch.

"It is one of the most prominent doctrines of Raja Yoga that the power of expelling thoughts, or if need be, killing them dead on the spot, *must* be attained. Naturally the art requires practice, but like other arts, when once acquired there is no mystery or difficulty about it. And it is worth practice. It may indeed fairly be said that life only begins when this art has been acquired. For obviously when instead of being ruled by individual thoughts, the whole flock of them in their immense multitude and variety and capacity is ours to direct and dispatch and employ where we list ('for He maketh the winds his messengers and the flaming fire His minister'), life becomes a thing so vast and grand compared with what it was before, that its former condition may well appear almost antenatal.

"If you can kill a thought dead, for the time being, you can do anything else with it that you please. And therefore, it is that this power is so valuable. And it not only frees a man from mental torment (which is nine-tenths at least of the torment of life), but it gives him a concentrated power of handling mental work absolutely unknown to him before. The two things are co-relative to each other. As already said, this is one of the principles of Raja Yoga.

"While at work your thought is to be absolutely concentrated in it, undistracted by anything whatever irrelevant to the matter in hand—pounding away like a great engine, with giant power and perfect economy—no wear and tear of friction, or dislocation of parts owing to the working of different forces at the same time. Then when the work is finished, if there is no more occasion for the use of the machine, it must stop equally, absolutely—stop entirely—no *worrying* (as if a parcel of boys were allowed to play their devilments with a locomotive as soon as it was in the shed)—and the man must retire into that region of his consciousness where his true self dwells.

"I say the power of the thought-machine itself is enormously increased by this faculty of letting it alone on the one hand, and of using it singly and with concentration on the other. It becomes a true tool, which a master-workman lays down when done with, but which only a bungler carries about with him all the time to show that he is the possessor of it."

We ask the students to read carefully the above quotations from Mr. Carpenter's book, for they are full of suggestions that may be taken up to advantage by those who are emancipating themselves from their slavery to the unmastered mind, and who are now bringing the mind under control of the Ego, by means of the Will.

Our next lesson will take up the subject of the relationship of the "I" to the Universal "I," and will be called the "Expansion of the Self." It will deal with the subject, not from a theoretical standpoint, but from the position of the teacher who is endeavoring to make his students actually *aware* in their consciousness of the truth of the proposition. In this course we are not trying to make our students past-masters of *theory*, but are endeavoring to place them in a position whereby they may *know* for themselves, and actually experience the things of which we teach.

Therefore, we urge upon you not to merely rest content with reading this lesson, but, instead, to study and meditate upon the teachings mentioned under the head of "Mental Drill," until the distinctions stand out clearly in your mind, and until you not only *believe* them to be true, but actually are *conscious* of the "I" and its Mental Tools. Have patience and perseverance. The task may be difficult, but the reward is great. To become conscious of the greatness, majesty, strength and power of your real being is worth years of hard study. Do you not think so? Then study and practice hopefully, diligently and earnestly.

Peace be with you.

MANTRAMS (AFFIRMATIONS) FOR THE SECOND LESSON

"I" am an entity—my mind is my instrument of expression.

"I" exist independent of my mind, and am not dependent upon it for existence or being.

"I" am Master of my mind, not its slave.

"I" can set aside my sensations, emotions, passions, desires, intellectual faculties, and all the rest of my mental collection of tools, as "not I" things—and still there remains something—and that something is "I," which cannot be set aside by me, for it is my very self; my only self; my real self—"I." That which remains after all that may be set aside *is* set aside is the "I"—Myself—eternal, constant, unchangeable.

THE THIRD LESSON

THE EXPANSION OF THE SELF.

In the first two lessons of this course, we have endeavored to bring to the candidate a realization in consciousness of the reality of the "I," and to enable him to distinguish between the Self and its sheaths, physical and mental. In the present lesson we will call his attention to the relationship of the "I" to the Universal "I," and will endeavor to give him an idea of a greater, grander Self, transcending personality and the little self that we are so apt to regard as the "I."

The keynote of this lesson will be "The Oneness of All," and all of its teachings will be directed to awakening a realization in consciousness of that great truth. But we wish to impress upon the mind of the Candidate that we are *not* teaching him that he is the Absolute. We are not teaching the "I Am God" belief, which we consider to be erroneous and misleading, and a perversion of the original Yogi teachings.

This false teaching has taken possession of many of the Hindu teachers and people, and with its accompanying teaching of "Maya" or the complete illusion or non-existence of the Universe, has reduced millions of people to a passive, negative mental condition which undoubtedly is retarding their progress. Not only in India is this true, but the same facts may be observed among the pupils of the Western teachers who have embraced this negative side of the Oriental Philosophy. Such people confound the "Absolute" and "Relative" aspects of the One, and, being unable to reconcile the facts of Life and the Universe with their theories of "I Am God," they are driven to the desperate expedient of boldly denying the Universe, and declaring it to be all "an illusion" or "Maya."

You will have no trouble in distinguishing the pupils of the teachers holding this view. They will be found to exhibit the most negative mental condition—a natural result of absorbing the constant suggestion of "nothingness"—the gospel of negation. In marked contrast to the mental condition of the students, however, will be observed the mental attitude of the teachers, who are almost uniformly examples of vital, positive, mental force, capable of hurling their teaching into the minds of the pupils—of driving in their statements by the force of an awakened Will. The teacher, as a rule, has awakened to a sense of the "I" consciousness, and really develops the same by his "I Am God" attitude, because by holding this mental attitude he is enabled to throw off the influence of the sheaths of the lower mental principles, and the light of the Self shows forth fiercely and strongly, sometimes to such an extent that it fairly scorches the mentality of the less advanced pupil. But, notwithstanding this awakened "I" consciousness, the teacher is handicapped by his intellectual misconception and befogging metaphysics, and is unable to impart the "I" consciousness to his pupils, and, instead of raising them up to shine with equal splendor with himself, he really forces them into a shadow by reason of his teachings.

Our students, of course, will understand that the above is not written in the spirit of carping criticism or fault-finding. We hold no such mental attitude, and indeed could not if we remain true to our conception of Truth. We are mentioning these matters simply that the student may avoid this "I Am God" pitfall which awaits the Candidate just as he has well started on the Path.

It would not be such a serious matter if it were merely a question of faulty metaphysics, for that would straighten itself out in time. But it is far more serious than this, for the teaching inevitably leads to the accompanying teaching that all is Illusion or *Maya*, and that Life is but a dream—a false thing—a lie—a nightmare; that the journey along the Path is but an illusion; that everything is "nothing"; that there is no soul; that You are God in disguise, and that He is fooling Himself in making believe that He is You; that Life is but a Divine masquerade or sleight-of-hand performance; that You are God, but that You (God) are fooling Yourself (God) in order to amuse Yourself (God). Is not this horrible?

And yet it shows to what lengths the human mind will go before it will part with some pet theory of metaphysics with which it has been hypnotized. Do you think that we have overdrawn the picture? Then read some of the teachings of these schools of the Oriental Philosophy, or listen to some of the more radical of the Western teachers preaching this philosophy. The majority of the latter lack the courage of the Hindu teachers in carrying their theories to a logical conclusion, and, consequently they veil their teachings with metaphysical subtlety. But a few of them are more courageous, and come out into the open and preach their doctrine in full.

Some of the modern Western teachers of this philosophy explain matters by saying that "God is masquerading as different forms of life, including Man, in order that he may gain the experience resulting therefrom, for although He has Infinite and Absolute Wisdom and Knowledge, he lacks the experience that comes only from actually living the life of the lowly forms, and therefore He descend thus in order to gain the needed experience."

Can you imagine the Absolute, possessed of all possible Knowledge and Wisdom, feeling the need of such petty "experience," and living the life of the lowly forms (including Man) in order "to gain experience?" To what Depths do these vain theories of Man drive us? Another leading Western teacher, who has absorbed the teaching of certain branches of the Oriental Philosophy, and who possesses the courage of his convictions, boldly announces that "You, yourself, are the *totality* of being, and with your mind alone create, preserve and destroy the universe, which is your own mental product."

And again, the last-mentioned teacher states: "the entire universe is a bagatelle illustration of your own creative power, which you are now exhibiting for your own inspection." "By their fruits shall you know them," is a safe rule to apply to all teachings. The philosophy that teaches that the Universe is an illusion perpetrated by you (God) to amuse, entertain or fool yourself (God), can have but one result, and that is the conclusion that "everything is nothing," and all that is necessary to do is to sit down, fold your hands and enjoy the Divine exhibition of legerdemain that you are performing for your own entertainment, and then, when the show is over, return to your state of conscious Godhood and recall with smiles the pleasant memories of the "conjure show" that you created to fool yourself with during several billions of ages.

That is what it amounts to, and the result is that those accepting this philosophy thrust upon them by forceful teachers, and knowing in their hearts that they are *not* God, but absorbing the suggestions of "nothingness," are driven into a state of mental apathy and negativity, the soul sinking into a stupor from which it may not be roused for a long period of time.

We wish you to avoid confounding our teaching with this just mentioned. We wish to teach you that You are a real Being—*not* God Himself, but a manifestation of Him who is the Absolute. You are a Child of the Absolute, if you prefer the term, possessed of the Divine Heritage, and whose mission it is to unfold qualities which are your inheritances from your Parent. Do not make the great mistake of confounding the Relative with the Absolute. Avoid this pitfall into which so many have fallen. Do not allow yourself to fall into the "Slough of Despond," and wallow in the mud of "nothingness," and to see no reality except in the person of some forceful teacher who takes the place of the Absolute in your mind. But raise your head and assert your Divine Parentage, and your Heritage from the Absolute, and step out boldly on the Path, asserting the "I."

(We must refer the Candidate back to our "Advanced Course," for our teachings regarding the Absolute and the Relative. The last three lessons of that course will throw light upon what we have just said To repeat the teaching at this point would be to use space which is needed for the lesson before us.)

And yet, while the "I" is *not* God, the Absolute, it is infinitely greater than we have imagined it to be before the light dawned upon us. It extends itself far beyond what we had conceived to be its limits. It touches the Universe at all its points, and is in the closest union with all of Life. It is in the closest touch with all that has emanated from the Absolute—all the world of Relativity. And while it faces the Relative Universe, it has its roots in the Absolute, and draws nourishment therefrom, just as does the babe in the womb obtain nourishment from the mother. It is verily a manifestation of God, and God's very essence is in it. Surely this is almost as "high" a statement as the "I Am God" of the teachers just mentioned, and yet how different. Let us consider the teaching in detail in this lesson, and in portions of others to follow.

Let us begin with a consideration of the instruments of the Ego, and the material with which and through which the Ego works. Let us realize that the physical body of man is identical in substance with all other forms of matter, and that its atoms are continually changing and being replaced, the material being drawn from the great storehouse of matter, and that there is a Oneness of matter underlying all apparent differences of form and substance. And then let us realize that the vital energy or *Prana* that man uses in his life work is but a portion of that great universal energy which permeates everything and everywhere, the portion being used by us at any particular moment being drawn from the universal supply, and again passing out from us into the great ocean of force or energy.

And then let us realize that even the mind, which is so close to the real Self that it is often mistaken for it—even that wonderful thing Thought—is but a portion of the Universal Mind, the highest emanation of the Absolute beneath the plane of Spirit, and that the Mind—substance or *Chitta* that we are using this moment, is not ours separately and distinctly, but is simply a portion from the great universal supply, which is constant and unchangeable. Let us then realize that even this thing that we feel pulsing within us—that which is so closely bound up with the Spirit as to be almost inseparable from it—that which we call Life—is but a bit of that Great Life Principle that pervades the Universe, and which cannot be added to, nor subtracted from.

When we have realized these things, and have begun to feel our relation (in these particulars) to the One Great Emanation of the Absolute, then we may begin to grasp the idea of the Oneness of Spirit, and the relation of the "I" to every other "I," and the merging of the Self into the one great Self, which is not the extinction of Individuality, as some have supposed, but the enlargement and extension of the Individual Consciousness until it takes in the Whole.

In Lessons X and XI, of the "Advanced Course" we called your attention to the Yogi teachings concerning *Akasa* or Matter, and showed you that all forms of what we know as Matter are but different forms of manifestation of the principle called *Akasa*, or as the Western scientists call it, "Ether." This Ether or *Akasa* is the finest, thinnest and most tenuous form of Matter, in fact it is Matter in its ultimate or fundamental form, the different forms of what we call Matter being but manifestations of this *Akasa* or Ether, the apparent difference resulting from different rates of vibration, etc.

We mention this fact here merely to bring clearly before your mind the fact of the Universality of Matter, to the end that you may realize that each and every particle of your physical body is but a portion of this great principle of the Universe, fresh from the great store-house, and just about returning to it again, for the atoms of the body are constantly changing. That which appears as your flesh to-day, may have been part of a plant a few days before, and may be part of some other living thing a few days hence. Constant change is going on, and what is yours to-day was someone's else yesterday, and still, another's to-morrow. You do not own one atom of matter *personally*, it is all a part of the common supply, the stream flowing through you and through all Life, on and on forever.

And so, it is with the Vital Energy that you are using every moment of your life. You are constantly drawing upon the great Universal supply of *Prana*, then using what is given you, allowing the force to pass on to assume some other form. It is the property of all, and all you can do is to use what you need, and allow it to pass on. There is but one Force or Energy, and that is to be found everywhere at all times.

And even the great principle, Mind-substance, is under the same law. It is hard for us to realize this. We are so apt to think of our mental operations as distinctively our own—something that belongs to us personally—that it is difficult for us to realize that Mind-substance is a Universal principle just as Matter or Energy, and that we are but drawing upon the Universal supply in our mental operations.

And more than this, the particular portion of Mind-substance that we are using, although separated from the Mind-substance used by other individuals by a thin wall of the very finest kind of Matter, is really in touch with the other apparently separated minds, and with the Universal Mind of which it forms a part. Just as is the Matter of which our physical bodies are composed really in touch with all Matter; and just as is the Vital Force used by us really in touch with all Energy; so is our Mind-substance really in touch with all Mind-substance. It is as if the Ego in its progress were moving through great oceans of Matter, Energy, or Mind-substance, making use of that of each which it needed and which immediately surrounded it, and leaving each behind as it moved on through the great volume of the ocean. This illustration is clumsy, but it may bring to your consciousness a realization that the Ego is the only thing that is really *Yours*, unchangeable and unaltered, and that all the rest is merely that portion of the Universal supply that you draw to yourself for the wants of the moment. It may also bring more clearly before your mind the great Unity of things—may enable you to see things as a Whole, rather than as separated parts. Remember, *You*—the "I"—are the only Real thing about and around you—all that has permanence—and Matter, Force and even Mind-substance, are but your instruments for use and expression. There are great oceans of each surrounding the "I" as it moves along.

It is well for you also to bear in mind the Universality of Life. All of the Universe is alive, vibrating and pulsating with life and energy and motion. There is nothing dead in the Universe. Life is everywhere, and always accompanied by intelligence. There is no such thing as a dead, unintelligent Universe. *Instead of being atoms of Life floating in a sea of death, we are atoms of Life surrounded by an ocean of Life, pulsating, moving, thinking, living.* Every atom of what we call Matter is alive. It has energy or force with it, and is always accompanied by intelligence and life. Look around us as we will—at the animal world—at the plant world—yes, even at the world of minerals and we see life, life, life—all alive and having intelligence. When we are able to bring this conception into the realm of actual consciousness—when we are able not only to intellectually accept this fact, but to even go still further and *feel* and be conscious of this Universal Life on all sides, then are we well on the road to attaining the Cosmic Consciousness.

But all these things are but steps leading up to the realization of the Oneness in Spirit, on the part of the Individual. Gradually there dawns upon him the realization that there is a Unity in the manifestation of Spirit from the Absolute—a unity with itself, and a Union with the Absolute. All this manifestation of Spirit on the part of the Absolute—all this begetting of Divine Children—was in the nature of a single act rather than as a series of acts, if we may be permitted to speak of the manifestation as an *act*.

Each Ego is a Centre of Consciousness in this great ocean of Spirit—each is a Real Self, apparently separate from the others and from its source, but the separation is only apparent in both cases, for there is the closest bond of union between the Egos of the Universe of Universes—each is knit to the other in the closest bond of union, and each is still attached to the Absolute by spiritual filaments, if we may use the term. In time we shall grow more conscious of this mutual relationship, as the sheaths are outgrown and cast aside, and in the end, we will be withdrawn into the Absolute—shall return to the Mansion of the Father.

It is of the highest importance to the developing soul to unfold into a realization of this relationship and unity, *for when this conception is once fully established the soul is enabled to rise above certain of the lower planes, and is free from the operation of certain laws that bind the undeveloped soul.*

Therefore, the Yogi teachers are constantly leading the Candidates toward this goal. First by this path, and then by that one, giving them different glimpses of the desired point, until finally the student finds a path best fitted for his feet, and he moves along straight to the mark, and throwing aside the confining bonds that have proved so irksome, he cries aloud for joy at his new found Freedom.

The following exercises and Mental Drills are intended to aid the Candidate in his work of growing into a realization of his relationship with the Whole of Life and Being.

MENTAL DRILL

(1) Read over what we have said in the "Advanced Course" regarding the principle known as Matter. Realize that all Matter is One at the last—that the real underlying substance of Matter is *Akasa* or Ether, and that all the varying forms evident to our senses are but modifications and grosser forms of that underlying principle. Realize that by known chemical processes all forms of Matter known to us, or rather all combinations resulting in "forms," may be resolved into their original elements, and that these elements are merely *Akasa* in different states of vibration. Let the idea of the Oneness of the visible Universe sink deeply into your mind, until it becomes fixed there. The erroneous conception of diversity in the material world must be replaced by the consciousness of Unity—Oneness, at the last, in spite of the appearance of variety and manifold forms. You must grow to see behind the world of forms of Matter, and see the great principle of Matter (*Akasa* or Ether) back of, within, and under it all. You must grow to *feel* this, as well as to intellectually see it.

(2) Meditate over the last-mentioned truths, and then follow the matter still further. Read what we have said in the "Advanced Course" (Lesson XI) about the last analysis of Matter showing it fading away into Force or Energy until the dividing line is lost, and Matter merges into Energy or Force, showing them both to be but the same thing, Matter being a grosser form of Energy or Force. This idea should be impressed upon the understanding, in order that the complete edifice of the Knowing of the Oneness may be complete in all of its parts.

(3) Then read in the "Advanced Lessons" about Energy or Force, in the oneness underlying its various manifestations. Consider how one form of Energy may be transformed into another, and so on around the circle, the one principle producing the entire chain of appearances. Realize that the energy within you by which you move and act, is but one of the forms of this great Principle of Energy with which the Universe is filled, and that you may draw to you the required Energy from the great Universal supply. But above all endeavor to grasp the idea of the Oneness pervading the world of Energy or Force, or Motion. See it in its entirety, rather than in its apparent separateness. These steps may appear somewhat tedious and useless, but take our word for it, they are all helps in fitting the mind to grasp the idea of the Oneness of All. Each step is important, and renders the next higher one more easily attained. In this mental drill, it will be well to mentally picture the Universe in perpetual motion—everything is in motion—all matter is moving and changing its forms, and manifesting the Energy within it. Suns and worlds rush through space, their particles constantly changing and moving. Chemical composition and decomposition is constant and unceasing, everywhere the work of building up and breaking down is going on. New combinations of atoms and worlds are constantly being formed and dissolved. And after considering this Oneness of the principle of Energy, reflect that through all these changes of form the Ego—the Real Self—YOU—stand unchanged and unharmed—Eternal, Invincible, Indestructible, Invulnerable, *Real* and Constant among this changing world of forms and force. You are above it all, and it revolves around and about you—Spirit.

(4) Read what we have said in the "Advanced Course" about Force or Energy, shading into Mind-substance which is its parent. Realize that Mind is back of all this great exhibition of Energy and Force that you have been considering. Then will you be ready to consider the Oneness of Mind.

(5) Read what we have said in the "Advanced Lessons" about Mind-substance. Realize that there is a great world of Mind-substance, or an Universal Mind, which is at the disposal of the Ego. All Thought is the product of the Ego's use of this Mind-substance, its tool and instrument. Realize that this Ocean of Mind is entire and Whole, and that the Ego may draw freely from it. Realize that *You* have this great ocean of Mind at your command, when you unfold sufficiently to use it. Realize that Mind is back of and underneath all of the world of form and names and action, and that in that sense: "All is Mind," although still higher in the scale than even Mind are *You*, the Real Self, the Ego, the Manifestation of the Absolute.

(6) Realize your identity with and relationship to All of Life. Look around you at Life in all its forms, from the lowest to the highest, all being exhibitions of the great

principle of Life in operation along different stages of The Path. Scorn not the humblest forms, but look behind the form and see the reality—Life. Feel yourself a part of the great Universal Life. Let your thought sink to the depths of the ocean, and realize your kinship with the Life back of the forms dwelling there. Do not confound the forms (often hideous from your personal point of view) with the principle behind them. Look at the plant-life, and the animal life, and seek to see behind the veil of form into the real Life behind and underneath the form. Learn to feel your Life throbbing and thrilling with the Life Principle in these other forms, and in the forms of those of your own race. Gaze into the starry skies and see there the numerous suns and worlds, all peopled with life in some of its myriad forms, and feel your kinship to it. If you can grasp this thought and consciousness, you will find yourself at-one-ment with those whirling worlds, and, instead of feeling small and insignificant by comparison, you will be conscious of an expansion of Self, until you feel that in those circling worlds is a part of yourself—that You are there also, while standing upon the Earth—that you are akin to all parts of the Universe—nay, more, that they are as much your home as is the spot upon which you are standing. You will find sweeping upon you a sense of consciousness that the Universe is your home— not merely a part of it, as you had previously thought. You will experience a sense of greatness, and broadness and grandness such as you have never dreamed of. You will begin to realize at least a part of your Divine inheritance, and to know indeed that you are a Child of the Infinite, the very essence of your Divine Parent being in the fibers of your being, At such times of realization one becomes conscious of what lies before the soul in its upward path, and how small the greatest prizes that Earth has to offer are when compared to some of these things before the soul, as seen by the eyes of the Spiritual Mind in moments of clear vision.

You must not dispute with these visions of the greatness of the soul, but must treat them hospitably, for they are your very own, coming to you from the regions of your Spiritual Mind which are unfolding into consciousness.

(7) The highest step in this dawning consciousness of the Oneness of All, is the one in which is realized that there is but One Reality, and at the same time the sense of consciousness that the "I" is in that Reality. It is most difficult to express this thought in words for it is something that must be felt, rather than seen by the Intellect. When the Soul realizes that the Spirit within it is, at the last, the only *real* part of it, and that the Absolute and its manifestation as Spirit is the only *real* thing in the Universe, a great step has been taken. But there is still one higher step to be taken before the full sense of the Oneness and Reality comes to us. That step is the one in which we realize the Identity of the "I" with the great "I" of the Universe. The mystery of the manifestation of the Absolute in the form of the

Spirit, is veiled from us—the mind confesses its inability to penetrate behind the veil shielding the Absolute from view, although it will give us a report of its being conscious of the presence of the Absolute just at the edge of the boundary line. But the highest region of the Spiritual Mind, when explored by the advanced souls who are well along the Path, reports that it sees beyond the apparent separation of Spirit from Spirit, and realizes that there is but one Reality of Spirit, and that all the "I"'s are really but different views of that One—Centers of Consciousness upon the surface of the One Great "I," the Centre of which is the Absolute Itself. This certainly penetrates the whole region of the Spiritual Mind, and gives us all the message of Oneness of the Spirit, just as the Intellect satisfies us with its message of the Oneness of Matter, Energy, and Mind. The idea of Oneness permeates all planes of Life.

The sense of Reality of the "I" that is apparent to You in the moments of your clearest mental vision, is really the reflection of the sense of Reality underlying the Whole—it is the consciousness of the Whole, manifesting through your point or Centre of Consciousness. The advanced student or Initiate finds his consciousness gradually enlarging until it realizes its identity with the Whole. He realizes that under all the forms and names of the visible world, there is to be found One Life—One Force—One Substance—One Existence—One Reality—ONE. And, instead of his experiencing any sense of the loss of identity or individuality, he becomes conscious of an enlargement of an expansion of individuality or identity—instead of feeling himself absorbed in the Whole, he feels that he is spreading out and embracing the Whole. This is most hard to express in words, for there are no words to fit the conception, and all that we can hope to do is to start into motion, by means of our words, the vibrations that will find a response in the minds of those who read the words, to the end that they will experience the consciousness which will bring its own understanding. This consciousness cannot be transmitted by words proceeding from the Intellect, but vibrations may be set up that will prepare the mind to receive the message from its own higher planes.

Even in the early stages of this dawning consciousness, one is enabled to identify the *real* part of himself with the *real* part of all the other forms of life that pass before his notice. In every other man—in every animal—in every plant—in every mineral—he sees behind the sheath and form of appearance, an evidence of the presence of the Spirit which is akin to his own Spirit—yea, more than akin, for the two are One. He sees Himself in all forms of life, in all time in all places. He realizes that the Real Self is everywhere present and everlasting, and that the Life within himself is also within all the Universe—in everything, for there is nothing dead in the Universe, and all Life, in all of its varying phases, is simply the One Life, held, used and enjoyed in common by all. Each Ego is a Centre of Consciousness in this great ocean of Life, and while apparently separate and distinct, is yet really in touch with the Whole, and with every apparent part.

It is not our intention, in this lesson, to go into the details of this great mystery of Life, or to recite the comparatively little of the Truth that the most advanced teachers and Masters have handed down. This is not the place for it—it belongs to the subject of Gnani Yoga rather than to Raja Yoga—and we touch upon it here, not for the purpose of trying to explain the scientific side of it to you, but merely in order that your minds may be led to take up the idea and gradually manifest it in conscious realization.

There is quite a difference between the scientific, intellectual teaching of Gnani Yoga, whereby the metaphysical and scientific sides of the Yogi teachings are presented to the minds of the students, in a logical, scientific manner, and the methods of Raja Yoga, in which the Candidate is led by degrees to a *consciousness* (outside of mere intellectual belief) of his real nature and powers. We are following the latter plan, for this course is a Course in *Raja* Yoga. We are aiming to present the matter to the mind in such a manner that it may prepare the way for the dawning consciousness, by brushing away the preconceived notions and prejudices, and allowing a clean entrance for the new conception.

Much that we have said in this lesson may appear, on the one hand, like useless repetition, and, on the other hand, like an incomplete presentation of the scientific side of the Yogi teachings. But it will be found, in time, that the effect has been that the mind of the student has undergone a change from the absorbing of the idea of the Oneness of Life, and the Expansion of the Self. The Candidate is urged not to be in too much of a hurry. Development must not be forced. Read what we have written, and practice the Mental Drills we have given, even if they may appear trifling and childish to some of you—we know what they will do for you, and you will agree with us in time. Make haste slowly. You will find that the mind will work out the matter, even though you be engaged in your ordinary work, and have forgotten the subject for the time. The greater portion of mental work is done in this way, while you are busy with something else, or even asleep, for the sub-conscious portion of the mind works along the lines pointed out for it, and performs its task.

As we have said, the purpose of this lesson is to bring you in the way of the unfoldment of consciousness, rather than to teach you the details of the scientific side of the Yogi teachings. Development is the keynote of Raja Yoga. And the reason that we wish to develop this sense of the Reality of the "I," and the Expansion of the Self, at this place is that thereby you may assert your Mastery over Matter, Energy and Mind. Before you may mount your throne as King, you must fully realize in consciousness that you *are* the *Reality* in this world of appearances. You must realize that you—the *real* You—are not only existent, and real, but that you are in touch with all else that is real, and that the roots of your being are grounded in the Absolute itself. You must realize that instead of being a separate atom of Reality, isolated and fixed in a narrow space, you are a Centre of Consciousness in the Whole of Reality, and that the Universe of Universes is your home—that your Centre of Consciousness might be moved on to a point trillions of miles from the Earth (which distance would be as nothing in Space) and still you—the awakened soul—would be just as much at home there as here—that even while you are here, your influence extends far out into space. Your real state, which will be revealed to you, gradually, throughout the ages, is so great and grand, that your mind in its present state of development cannot grasp even the faint reflection of that glory.

We wish you to try to form at least a faint idea of your Real State of Being, in order that you may control the lower principles by the force of your awakened Will, which Will depends upon your degree of consciousness of the Real Self.

As man grows in understanding and consciousness of the Real Self, so does his ability to use his Will grow. Will is the attribute of the Real Self. It is well that this great realization of the Real Self brings with it Love for all of Life, and Kindness, for, were it not so, the Will that comes to him who grows into a realization of his real being could be used to the great hurt of those of the race who had not progressed so far (their *relative* hurt, we mean, for in the end, and at the last, no soul is ever really *hurt*). But the dawning power brings with it greater Love and Kindness, and the higher the soul mounts the more is it filled with the higher ideals and the more does it throw from it the lower animal attributes.

It is true that some souls growing into a consciousness of their real nature, without an understanding of what it all means, may commit the error of using the awakened Will for selfish ends, as may be seen in the cases of the Black Magicians spoken of in the occult writings, and also in the cases of well-known characters in history and in modern life, who manifest an enormous Will which they misuse. All of this class of people of great Will have stumbled or grown blindly into a consciousness (or partial consciousness) of the real nature, but lack the restraining influence of the higher teachings. But such misuse of the Will brings pain and unrest to the user, and he is eventually driven into the right road.

We do not expect our students to grasp fully this idea of the Expansion of Self. Even the highest grasp it only partially. But until you get a glimmering of the consciousness you will not be able to progress far on the path of Raja Yoga. You must understand *what you are*, before you are able to use the power that lies dormant within you. You must realize that you are the Master, before you can claim the powers of the Master, and expect to have your commands obeyed. So bear patiently with us, your Teachers, while we set before you the lessons to be learned—the tasks to be performed. The road is long, and is rough in places—the feet may become tired and bruised, but the reward is great, and there are resting places along the path. Be not discouraged if your progress seems slow, for the soul must unfold naturally as does the flower, without haste, without force.

And be not dismayed nor affrighted if you occasionally catch a glimpse of your higher self. As "M.C." says, in her notes on "Light on the Path" (see "Advanced Course," page 95): "To have seen thy soul in its bloom, is to have obtained a momentary glimpse in thyself of the transfiguration which shall eventually make thee more than man; to recognize, is to achieve the great task of gazing upon the blazing light without dropping the eyes, and not falling back in terror as though before some ghastly phantom. This happens to some, and so, when the victory is all but won, it is lost."

Peace be with thee.

MANTRAM (AFFIRMATION) FOR THE THIRD LESSON

There is but one ultimate form of Matter; one ultimate form of Energy; one ultimate form of Mind. Matter proceeds from Energy, and Energy from Mind, and all are an emanation of the Absolute, threefold in appearance but One in substance. There is but One Life, and that permeates the Universe, manifesting in various forms, but being, at the last, but One. My body is one with Universal Matter; My energy and vital force is one with the Universal Energy; My Mind is one with the Universal Mind; My Life is one with the Universal Life. The Absolute has expressed and manifested itself in Spirit, which is the real "I" overshadowing and embracing all the apparently separate "I"s. "I" feel my identity with Spirit and realize the Oneness of All Reality. I feel my unity with all Spirit, and my Union (through Spirit) with the Absolute. I realize that "I" am an Expression and Manifestation of the Absolute, and that its very essence is within me. I am filled with Divine Love. I am filled with Divine Power. I am filled with Divine Wisdom. I am conscious of identity in spirit, in substance; and in nature; with the One Reality.

THE FOURTH LESSON

MENTAL CONTROL.

In our first three lessons of this series, we have endeavored to bring into realization within your mind (1) the consciousness of the "I"; its independence from the body; its immortality; its invincibility and invulnerability; (2) the superiority of the "I" over the mind, as well as over the body; the fact that the mind is not the "I," but is merely an instrument for the expression of the "I"; the fact that the "I" is master of the mind, as well as of the body; that the "I" is behind all thought; that the "I" can set aside for consideration the sensations, emotions, passions, desires, and the rest of the mental phenomena, and still realize that it, the "I," is apart from these mental manifestations, and remains unchanged, real and fully existent; that the "I" can set aside any and all of its mental tools and instruments, as "not I" things, and still consciously realize that after so setting them aside there remains something—itself—the "I" which cannot be set aside or taken from; that the "I" is the master of the mind, and not its slave; (3) that the "I" is a much greater thing than the little personal "I" we have been considering it to be; that the "I" is a part of that great One Reality which pervades all the Universe; that it is connected with all other forms of life by countless ties, mental and spiritual filaments and relations; that the "I" is a Centre of Consciousness in that great One Reality or Spirit, which is behind and back of all Life and Existence, the Centre of which Reality or Existence, is the Absolute or God; that the sense of Reality that is inherent in the "I," is really the reflection of the sense of Reality inherent in the Whole—the Great "I" of the Universe.

The underlying principle of these three lessons is the Reality of the "I," in itself, over and above all Matter, Force, or Mind—positive to all of them, just as they are positive or negative to each other—and negative only to the Centre of the One—the Absolute itself. And this is the position for the Candidate or Initiate to take: "I am positive to Mind, Energy, and Matter, and control them all—I am negative only to the Absolute, which is the Centre of Being, of which Being I Am. And, as I assert my mastery over Mind, Energy, and Matter, and exercise my Will over them, so do I acknowledge my subordination to the Absolute, and gladly open my soul to the inflow of the Divine Will, and partake of its Power, Strength, and Wisdom."

In the present lesson, and those immediately following it, we shall endeavor to assist the Candidate or Initiate in acquiring a mastery of the subordinate manifestations, Matter, Energy, and Mind. In order to acquire and assert this mastery, one must acquaint himself with the nature of the thing to be controlled.

In our "Advanced Course" we have endeavored to explain to you the nature of the Three Great Manifestations, known as *Chitta*, or Mind-Substance; *Prana*, or Energy; and *Akasa*, or the Principle of Matter. We also explained to you that the "I" of man is superior to these three, being what is known as *Atman* or Spirit. Matter, Energy, and Mind, as we have explained, are manifestations of the Absolute, and are relative things.

The Yogi philosophy teaches that Matter is the grossest form of manifested substance, being below Energy and Mind, and consequently negative to, and subordinate to both. One stage higher than Matter, is Energy or Force, which is positive to, and has authority over, Matter (Matter being a still grosser form of substance), but which is negative to and subordinate to Mind, which is a still higher form of substance. Next in order comes the highest of the three—Mind—the finest form of substance, and which dominates both Energy and Matter, being positive to both. Mind, however is negative and subordinate to the "I," which is Spirit, and obeys the orders of the latter when firmly and intelligently given. The "I" itself is subordinate only to the Absolute—the Centre of Being—the "I" being positive and dominant over the threefold manifestation of Mind, Energy, and Matter.

The "I," which for the sake of the illustration must be regarded as a separate thing (although it is really only a Centre of Consciousness in the great body of Spirit), finds itself surrounded by the triple-ocean of Mind, Energy and Matter, which ocean extends into Infinity. The body is but a physical form through which flows an unending stream of matter, for, as you know the particles and atoms of the body are constantly changing; being renewed; replaced; thrown off, and supplanted. One's body of a few years ago, or rather the particles composing that body, have passed off and now form new combinations in the world of matter.

And one's body of to-day is passing away and being replaced by new particles. And one's body of next year is now occupying some other portion of space, and its particles are now parts of countless other combinations, from which space and combinations they will later come to combine and form the body of next year. There is nothing permanent about the body—even the particles of the bones are being constantly replaced by others. And so, it is with the Vital Energy, Force, or Strength of the body (including that of the brain). It is constantly being used up, and expended, a fresh supply taking its place. And even the Mind of the person is changeable, and the Mind-substance or *Chitta*, is being used up and replenished, the new supply coming from the great Ocean of Mind, into which the discarded portion slips, just as is the case with the matter and energy.

While the majority of our students, who are more or less familiar with the current material scientific conceptions, will readily accept the above idea of the ocean of Matter, and Energy, and the fact that there is a continual using up and replenishing of one's store of both, they may have more or less trouble in accepting the idea that Mind is a substance or principle amenable to the same general laws as are the other two manifestations, or attributes of substance. One is so apt to think of his Mind as "himself"—the "I." Notwithstanding the fact that in our Second Lesson of this series we showed you that the "I" is superior to the mental states, and that it can set them aside and regard and consider them as "not-I" things, yet the force of the habit of thought is very strong, and it may take some of you considerable time before you "get into the way" of realizing that your Mind is "something that you use," instead of being You—yourself.

And yet, you must persevere in attaining this realization, for in the degree that you realize your dominance over your mind, so will be your control of it, and its amenability to that control. And, as is the degree of that dominance and control, so will be the character, grade and extent of the work that your Mind will do for you. So, you see: *Realization brings Control—and Control brings results*. This statement lies at the base of the science of *Raja Yoga*. And many of its first exercises are designed to acquaint the student with that realization, and to develop the realization and control by habit and practice.

The Yogi Philosophy teaches that instead of Mind being the "I." it is the thing through and by means of which the "I" *thinks*, at least so far as is concerned the knowledge concerning the phenomenal or outward Universe—that is the Universe of Name and Form. There is a higher Knowledge locked up in the innermost part of the "I," that far transcends any information that it may receive about or from the outer world, but that is not before us for consideration at this time, and we must concern ourselves with the "thinking" about the world of things.

Mind-substance in Sanskrit is called "*Chitta*," and a wave in the *Chitta* (which wave is the combination of Mind and Energy) is called "*Vritta*," which is akin to what we call a "thought." In other words, it is "mind in action," whereas *Chitta* is "mind in repose." *Vritta*, when literally translated means "a whirlpool or eddy in the mind," which is exactly what a thought really is.

But we must call the attention of the student, at this point, to the fact that the word "Mind" is used in two ways by the Yogis and other occultists, and the student is directed to form a clear conception of each meaning, in order to avoid confusion, and that he may more clearly perceive the two aspects of the things which the word is intended to express. In the first place the word "Mind" is used as synonymous with *Chitta*, or Mind-substance, which is the Universal Mind Principle. From this *Chitta*, Mind-substance, or Mind, all the material of the millions of personal minds is obtained. The second meaning of the word "Mind" is that which we mean when we speak of the "mind" of anyone, thereby meaning the mental faculties of that particular person—that which distinguishes his mental personality from that of another.

We have taught you that this "mind" in Man, functions on three planes, and have called the respective manifestations (1) the Instinctive Mind; (2) the Intellect; and (3) the Spiritual Mind. (*See "Fourteen Lessons in Yogi Philosophy," etc.*) These three mental planes, taken together, make up the "mind" of the person, or to be more exact they, clustered around the "I" form the "soul" of the individual. The word "soul" is often used as synonymous with "spirit" but those who have followed us will distinguish the difference. The "soul" is the Ego surrounded by its mental principles, while the Spirit is the "soul of the soul"—the "I," or Real Self.

The Science of *Raja Yoga*, to which this series of lessons is devoted, teaches, as its basic principle, the Control of the Mind. It holds that the first step toward Power consists in obtaining a control of one's own mind. It holds that the internal world must be conquered before the outer world is attacked. It holds that the "I" manifests itself in Will, and that that Will may be used to manipulate, guide, govern and direct the mind of its owner, as well as the physical world. It aims to clear away all mental rubbish, and encumbrances—to conduct a "mental house-cleaning," as it were, and to secure a clear, clean, healthy mind. Then it proceeds to control that mind intelligently, and with effect, saving all waste-power, and by means of concentration bringing the Mind in full harmony with the Will, that it may be brought to a focus and its power greatly increased and its efficiency fully secured.

Concentration and Will-power are the means by which the Yogis obtain such wonderful results, and by which they manage and direct their vigorous, healthy minds, and master the material world, acting positively upon Energy and Matter. This control extends to all planes of the Mind and the Yogis not only control the Instinctive Mind, holding in subjection its lower qualities and making use of its other parts, but they also develop and enlarge the field of their Intellect and obtain from it wonderful results. Even the Spiritual Mind is mastered, and aided in its unfoldment, and urged to pass down into the field of consciousness some of the wonderful secrets to be found within its area.

By means of *Raja Yoga* many of the secrets of existence and Being—many of the Riddles of the Universe—are answered and solved. And by it the latent powers inherent in the constitution of Man are unfolded and brought into action. Those highly advanced in the science are believed to have obtained such a wonderful degree of power and control over the forces of the universe, that they are as gods compared with the ordinary man.

Raja Yoga teaches that not only may power of this kind be secured, but that a wonderful field of Knowledge is opened out through its practice. It holds that when the concentrated mind is focused upon thing or subject, the true nature and inner meaning, of, and concerning, that thing or subject will be brought to view. The concentrated mind passes through the object or subject just as the X-Ray passes through a block of wood, and the thing is seen by the "I" as it *is*—in truth—and not as it had appeared before, imperfectly and erroneously. Not only may the outside world be thus explored, but the mental ray may be turned inward, and the secret places of the mind explored. When it is remembered that the bit of mind that each man possesses, is like a drop of the ocean which contains within its tiny compass all the elements that make up the ocean, and that to know perfectly the drop is to know perfectly the ocean, then we begin to see what such a power really means.

Many in the Western world who have attained great results in the intellectual and scientific fields of endeavor, have developed these powers more or less unconsciously. Many great inventors are practical Yogis, although they do not realize the source of their power. Anyone who is familiar with the personal mental characteristics of Edison, will see that he follows some of the *Raja Yoga* methods, and that Concentration is one of his strongest weapons.

And from all reports, Prof. Elmer Gates, of Washington, D.C., whose mind has unfolded many wonderful discoveries and inventions, is also a practical Yogi although he may repudiate the assertion vigorously, and may not have familiarized himself with the principles of this science, which he has "dropped into" unconsciously. Those who have reported upon Prof. Gates' methods, say that he fairly "digs out" the inventions and discoveries from his mind, after going into seclusion and practicing concentration, and what is known as the Mental Vision.

But we have given you enough of theory for one lesson, and must begin to give you directions whereby you may aid yourself in developing these latent powers and unfolding these dormant energies. You will notice that in this series we first tell you something about the theory, and then proceed to give you "something to do." This is the true Yogi method as followed and practiced by their best teachers. Too much theory is tiresome, and sings the mind to sleep, while too much exercise tires one, and does not give the inquiring part of his mind the necessary food. To combine both in suitable proportions is the better plan, and one that we aim to follow.

MENTAL DRILL AND EXERCISES

Before we can get the mind to do good work for us, we must first "tame" it, and bring it to obedience to the Will of the "I." The mind, as a rule, has been allowed to run wild, and follow its own sweet will and desires, without regard to anything else. Like a spoiled child or badly trained domestic animal, it gets into much trouble, and is of very little pleasure, comfort or use. The minds of many of us are like menageries of wild animals, each pursuing the bent of its own nature, and going its own way. We have the whole menagerie within us—the tiger, the ape, the peacock, the ass, the goose, the sheep the hyena, and all the rest. And we have been letting these animals rule us. Even our Intellect is erratic, unstable, and like the quicksilver to which the ancient occultists compared it, shifting and uncertain. If you will look around you, you will see that those men and women in the world who have really accomplished anything worthwhile have trained their minds to obedience. They have asserted the Will over their own minds, and learned Mastery and Power in that way. The average mind chafes at the restraint of the Will, and is like a frisky monkey that will not be "taught tricks." But taught it must be, if it wants to do good work. And teach it you must if you expect to get any use from it—if you expect to use it, instead of having it use you.

And this is the first thing to be learned in *Raja Yoga*—this control of the mind. Those who had hoped for some royal road to mastery, may be disappointed, but there is only one way and that is to master and control the mind by the Will. Otherwise, it will run away when you most need it. And so we shall give you some exercise designed to aid you in this direction.

The first exercise in *Raja Yoga* Is what is called *Pratyahara* or the art of making the mind introspective or turned inward upon itself. It is the first step toward mental control. It aims to turn the mind from going outward, and gradually turning it inward upon itself or inner nature. The object is to gain control of it by the Will. The following exercises will aid in that direction:

EXERCISE I.

(a) Place yourself in a comfortable position, and so far, as possible free from outside disturbing influences. Make no violent effort to control the mind, but rather allow it to run along for a while and exhaust its efforts. It will take advantage of the opportunity, and will jump around like an unchained monkey at first, until it gradually slows down and looks to you for orders. It may take some time to tame down at first trial, but each time you try it will come around to you in shorter time.

The Yogis spend much time in acquiring this mental peace and calm, and consider themselves well paid for it.

(b) When the mind is well calmed down, and peaceful, fix the thought on the "I Am," as taught in our previous lessons. Picture the "I" as an entity independent of the body; deathless; invulnerable; immortal; real. Then think of it as independent of the body, and able to exist without its fleshly covering. Meditate upon this for a time, and then gradually direct the thought to the realization of the "I" as independent and superior to the mind, and controlling same. Go over the general ideas of the first two lessons, and endeavor to calmly reflect upon them and to see them in the "mind's eye." You will find that your mind is gradually becoming more and more peaceful and calm, and that the distracting thoughts of the outside world are farther and farther removed from you.

(c) Then let the mind pass on to a calm consideration of the Third Lesson, in which we have spoken of the Oneness of All, and the relationship of the "I" to the One Life; Power; Intelligence; Being. You will find that you are acquiring a mental control and calm heretofore unknown to you. The exercises in the first three lessons will have prepared you for this.

(d) The following is the most difficult of the variations or degrees of this exercise, but the ability to perform it will come gradually. The exercise consists in gradually shutting out all thought or impression of the outside world; of the body; and of the thoughts themselves, the student concentrating and meditating upon the word and idea "I AM," the idea being that he shall concentrate upon the idea of mere "being" or "existence," symbolized by the words "I Am." Not "I am *this*," or "I am *that*," or "I *do* this," or "I *think* that," but simply: "I *AM*." This exercise will focus the attention at the very center of Being within oneself, and will gather in all the mental energies, instead of allowing them to be scattered upon outside things. A feeling of Peace, Strength, and Power will result, for the affirmation, and the thought back of it, is the most powerful and strongest that one may make, for it is a statement of Actual Being, and a turning of the thought inward to that truth. Let the mind first dwell upon the word "I," identifying it with the Self, and then let it pass on to the word "AM," which signifies Reality, and Being. Then combine the two with the meanings thereof, and the result a most powerful focusing of thought inward, and most potent Statement of Being.

It is well to accompany the above exercises with a comfortable and easy physical attitude, so as to prevent the distraction of the attention by the body. In order to do this one should assume an easy attitude and then relax every muscle, and take the tension from every nerve, until a perfect sense of ease, comfort and relaxation is obtained. You should practice this until you have fully acquired it. It will be useful to you in many ways, besides rendering Concentration and Meditation easier. It will act as a "rest cure" for tired body, nerves, and mind.

EXERCISE II.

The second step in *Raja Yoga* is what is known as *Dharana*, or Concentration. This is a most wonderful idea in the direction of focusing the mental forces, and may be cultivated to an almost incredible degree, but all this requires work, time, and patience. But the student will be well repaid for it. Concentration consists in the mind focusing upon a certain subject, or object, and being held there for a time. This, at first thought seems very easy, but a little practice will show how difficult it is to firmly fix the attention and hold it there. It will have a tendency to waver, and move to some other object or subject, and much practice will be needed in order to hold it at the desired point. But practice will accomplish wonders, as one may see by observing people who have acquired this faculty, and who use it in their everyday life. But the following point should be remembered. Many persons have acquired the faculty of concentrating their attention, but have allowed it to become almost involuntary, and they become a slave to it, forgetting themselves and everything else, and often neglecting necessary affairs.

This is the ignorant way of concentrating, and those addicted to it become slaves to their habits, instead of masters of their minds. They become day-dreamers, and absent-minded people, instead of Masters. They are to be pitied as much as those who cannot concentrate at all. The secret is in a mastery of the mind. The Yogis can concentrate at will, and completely bury themselves in the subject before them, and extract from it every item of interest, and can then pass the mind from the thing at will, the same control being used in both cases. They do not allow fits of abstraction, or "absent-mindedness" to come upon them, nor are they day-dreamers. On the contrary they are very wide-awake individuals; close observers; clear thinkers; correct reasoners. They are masters of their minds, not slaves to their moods. The ignorant concentrator buries himself in the object or subject, and allows it to master and absorb himself, while the trained Yogi thinker asserts the "I," and then directs his mind to concentrate upon the subject or object, keeping it well under control and in view all the time. Do you see the difference? Then heed the lesson.

The following exercises may be found useful in the first steps of Concentration:

(a) Concentrate the attention upon some familiar object—a pencil, for instance. Hold the mind there and consider the pencil to the exclusion of any other object.

Consider its size; color; shape; kind of wood. Consider its uses, and purposes; its materials; the process of its manufacture, etc., etc., etc. In short think as many things about the pencil as possible allowing the mind to pursue any associated by-paths, such as a consideration of the graphite of which the "lead" is made; the forest from which came the wood used in making the pencil; the history of pencils, and other implements used for writing, etc. In short exhaust the subject of "Pencils." In considering a subject under concentration, the following plan of synopsis will be found useful. Think of the thing in question from the following view-points:

(1) The thing itself.

(2) The place from whence it came.

(3) Its purpose or use.

(4) Its associations.

(5) Its probable end.

Do not let the apparently trivial nature of the inquiry discourage you, for the simplest form of mental training is useful, and will help to develop your Will and Concentration. It is akin to the process of developing a physical muscle by some simple exercise, and in both cases, one loses sight of the unimportance of the exercise itself, in view of the end to be gained.

(b) Concentrate the attention upon some part of the body—the hand for instance, and fixing your entire attention upon it, shut off or inhibit all sensation from the other parts of the body. A little practice will enable you to do this. In addition to the mental training, this exercise will stimulate the part of the body concentrated upon, for reasons that will appear in future lessons. Change the parts of the body concentrated upon, and thus give the mind a variety of exercises, and the body the effect of a general stimulation.

(c) These exercises may be extended indefinitely upon familiar objects about you. Remember always, that the thing in itself is of no importance, the whole idea being to train the mind to obey the Will, so that when you really wish to use the mental forces upon some important object, you may find them well trained and obedient. Do not be tempted to slight this part of the work because it is "dry" and uninteresting, for it leads up to things that are most interesting, and opens a door to a fascinating subject.

(d) Practice focusing the attention upon some abstract subject—that is upon some subject of interest that may offer a field for mental exploration. Think about the subject in all its phases and branches, following up one by-path, and then another, until you feel that you know all about the subject that your mind has acquired. You will be surprised to find how much more you know about any one thing or subject than you had believed possible. In hidden corners of your mind, you will find some useful or interesting information about the thing in question, and when you are through you will feel well posted upon it, and upon the things connected with it. This exercise will not only help, to develop your intellectual powers, but will strengthen your memory, and broaden your mind, and give you more confidence in yourself. And, in addition, you will have taken a valuable exercise in Concentration or *Dharana*.

The Importance of Concentration.

Concentration is a focusing of the mind. And this focusing of the mind requires a focusing, or bringing to a center, of the Will. The mind is concentrated because the Will is focused upon the object. The mind flows into the mold made by the Will. The above exercises are designed not only to accustom the mind to the obedience and direction of the Will, but also tend to accustom the Will to command. We speak of strengthening the Will, when what we really mean is training the mind to obey, and accustoming the Will to command. Our Will is strong enough, but we do not realize it. The Will takes root in the very center of our being—in the "I," but our imperfectly developed mind does not recognize this tact. We are like young elephants that do not recognize their own strength, but allow themselves to be mastered by puny drivers, whom they could brush aside with a movement. The Will is back of all action—all doing—mental and physical.

We shall have much to say touching the Will, in these lessons and the student should give the matter his careful attention. Let him look around him, and he will see that the great difference between the men who have stepped forward from the ranks, and those who remain huddled up in the crowd, consists in Determination and Will. As Buxton has well said: "The longer I live, the more certain I am that the great difference between men, the feeble and the powerful; the great and the insignificant; is Energy and Invincible Determination." And he might have added that the thing behind that "energy and invincible determination" was Will.

The writers and thinkers of all ages have recognized the wonderful and transcendent importance of the Will. Tennyson sings: "O living Will thou shalt endure when all that seems shall suffer shock." Oliver Wendell Holmes says: "The seat of the Will seems to vary with the organ through which it is manifested; to transport itself to different parts of the brain, as we may wish to recall a picture, a phrase, a melody; to throw its force on the muscles or the intellectual processes. Like the general-in-chief, its place is everywhere in the field of action. It is the least like an instrument of any of our faculties; the farthest removed from our conceptions of mechanism and matter, as we commonly define them." Holmes was correct in his idea, but faulty in his details. The Will does not change its seat, which is always in the center of the Ego, but the Will forces the mind to all parts, and in all directions, and it directs the *Prana* or vital force likewise. The Will is indeed the general-in-chief, but it does not rush to the various points of action, but sends its messengers and couriers there to carry out its orders. Buxton has said: "The Will will do anything that can be done in this world. And no talents, no circumstances, no opportunities will make a two-legged creature a Man without it." Ik Marvel truly says: "Resolve is what makes a man manifest; not puny resolve, not crude determinations, not errant purpose—but that strong and indefatigable Will which treads down difficulties and danger, as a boy treads down the heaving frost-lands of winter; which kindles his eye and brain with a proud pulse-beat toward the unattainable. Will makes men giants."

The great obstacle to the proper use of the Will, in the case of the majority of people, is the lack of ability to focus the attention. The Yogis clearly understand this point, and many of the *Raja Yoga* exercises which are given to the students by the teachers, are designed to overcome this difficulty. Attention is the outward evidence of the Will. As a French writer has said: "The attention is subject to the superior authority of the Ego. I yield it, or I withhold it, as I please. I direct it in turn to several points. I concentrate it upon each point as long as my Will can stand the effort." Prof. James has said: "The essential achievement of the Will, when it is most voluntary, is to attend to a difficult object, and hold it fast before the mind. Effort of Attention is the essential phenomenon of the Will."

And Prof. Halleck says: "The first step toward the development of Will lies in the exercise of Attention. Ideas grow in distinctness and motor-power as we attend to them. If we take two ideas of the same intensity and center the attention upon one, we shall notice how much it grows in power." Prof. Sully says: "Attention may be roughly defined as the active self-direction of the mind to any object which presents itself at the moment." The word "Attention" is derived from two Latin words, *ad tendere*, meaning "to stretch towards," and this is just what the Yogis know it to be. By means of their psychic or clairvoyant sight, they see the thought of the attentive person stretched out toward the object attended to, like a sharp wedge, the point of which is focused upon the object under consideration, the entire force of the thought being concentrated at that point. This is true not only when the person is considering an object, but when he is earnestly impressing his ideas upon another, or upon some task to be accomplished. Attention means reaching the mind out to and focusing it upon something.

The trained Will exhibits itself in a tenacious Attention, and this Attention is one of the signs of the trained Will. The student must not hastily conclude that this kind of Attention is a common faculty among men. On the contrary it is quite rare, and is seen only among those of "strong" mentality. Anyone may fasten his Attention upon some passing, *pleasing* thing, but it takes a trained will to fasten it upon some unattractive thing, and hold it there. Of course, the trained occultist is able to throw interest into the most unattractive thing upon which it becomes advisable to focus his Attention, but this, in itself, comes with the trained Will, and is not the possession of the average man. Voluntary Attention is rare, and is found only among strong characters. But it may be cultivated and grown, until he who has scarcely a shade of it to-day, in time may become a giant. It is all a matter of practice, exercise, and Will.

It is difficult to say too much in favor of the development of the faculty of tenacious Attention. One possessing this developed faculty is able to accomplish far more than even a much "brighter" man who lacks it. And the best way to train the Attention, under the direction of the Will, is to practice upon *uninteresting* objects, and ideas, holding them before the mind until they begin to assume an Interest.

This is difficult at first, but the task soon begins to take on a pleasant aspect, for one finds that his Will-power and Attention are growing, and he feels himself acquiring a Force and Power that were lacking before—he realizes that he is growing Stronger. Charles Dickens said that the secret of his success consisted in his developing a faculty of throwing his entire Attention into whatever he happened to be doing at the moment and then being able to turn that same degree of Attention to the next thing coming before him for consideration. He was like a man behind a great searchlight, which was successively turned upon point after point, illuminating each in turn. The "I" is the man behind the light, and the Will is the reflector, the light being the Attention.

This discussion of Will and Attention may seem somewhat "dry" to the student, but that is all the more reason that he should attend to it. It is the secret that lies at the basis of the Science of *Raja Yoga*, and the Yogi Masters have attained a degree of Concentrated Will and Attention that would be inconceivable to the average "man on the street." By reason of this, they are able to direct the mind here and there, outward or inward, with an enormous force. They are able to focus the mind upon a small thing with remarkable intensity, just as the rays of the sun may be focused through a "sun-glass" and caused to ignite linen, or, on the other hand, they are able to send forth the mind with intense energy, illuminating whatever it rests upon, just as happens in the case of the strong electric searchlight, with which many of us are familiar. By all means start in to cultivate the Attention and Will. Practice on the unpleasant tasks—do the things that you have before you, and from which you have been shrinking because they were unpleasant. Throw interest into them, and the difficulty will vanish, and you will come out of it much stronger, and filled with a new sense of Power.

MANTRAM (AFFIRMATION)

"I" have a Will—it is my inalienable property and right. I determine to cultivate and develop it by practice and exercise. My mind is obedient to my Will. I assert my Will over my Mind. I am Master of my mind and body. I *assert* my Mastery. My Will is Dynamic—full of Force and Energy, and Power. I feel my strength. I am Strong. I am Forceful. I am Vital. I am Center of Consciousness, Energy, Strength, and Power, and I claim my birthright.

THE FIFTH LESSON

THE CULTIVATION OF ATTENTION.

In our last lesson we called your attention to the fact that the Yogis devote considerable time and practice to the acquirement of Concentration. And we also had something to say regarding the relation of Attention to the subject of Concentration. In this lesson we shall have more to say on the subject of Attention, for it is one of the important things relating to the practice of *Raja Yoga*, and the Yogis insist upon their students practicing systematically to develop and cultivate the faculty. Attention lies at the base of Will-power, and the cultivation of one makes easy the exercise of the other.

To explain why we lay so much importance to the cultivation of Attention, would necessitate our anticipating future lessons of this series, which we do not deem advisable at this time. And so, we must ask our students to take our word for it, that all that we have to say regarding the importance of the cultivation of Attention, is occasioned by the relation of that subject to the use of the mind in certain directions as will appear fully later on.

In order to let you know that we are not advancing some peculiar theory of the Yogis, which may not be in harmony with modern Western Science, we give you in this article a number of quotations, from Western writers and thinkers, touching upon this important faculty of the mind, so that you may see that the West and East agree upon this main point, however different may be their explanations of the fact, or their use of the power gained by the cultivation of Attention.

As we said in our last lesson, the word Attention is derived from two Latin words "*ad tendere*," meaning "to stretch toward," which is really what Attention is. The "I" wills that the mind be focused on some particular object or thing, and the mind obeys and "stretches toward" that object or thing, focusing its entire energy upon it, observing every detail, dissecting, analyzing, consciously and sub-consciously, drawing to itself every possible bit of information regarding it, both from within and from without. We cannot lay too much stress upon the acquirement of this great faculty, or rather, the development of it, for it is necessary for the intelligent study of *Raja Yoga*.

In order to bring out the importance of the subject, suppose we start in by actually giving our Attention to the subject of Attention, and see how much more there is in it than we had thought. We shall be well repaid for the amount of time and trouble expended upon it.

Attention has been defined as a focusing of consciousness, or, if one prefers the form of expression, as "detention in consciousness." In the first case, we may liken it to the action of the sun-glass through which the sun's rays are concentrated upon an object, the result being that the heat is gathered together at a small given point, the intensity of the same being raised many degrees until the heat is sufficient to burn a piece of wood, or evaporate water. If the rays were not focused, the same rays and heat would have been scattered over a large surface, and the effect and power lessened. And so, it is with the mind. If it is allowed to scatter itself over the entire field of a subject, it will exert but little power and the results will be weak. But if it is passed through the sun-glass of attention, and focused first over one part, and then over another, and so on, the matter may be mastered in detail, and a result accomplished that will seem little less than marvelous to those who do not know the secret.

Thompson has said: "The experiences most permanently impressed upon consciousness, are those upon which the greatest amount of attention has been fixed."

Another writer upon the subject has said that "Attention is so essentially necessary to understanding, that without some degree of it the ideas and perceptions that pass through the mind seem to leave no trace behind them."

Hamilton has said: "An act of attention, that is, an act of concentration, seems thus necessary to every exertion of consciousness, as a certain contraction of the pupil is requisite to every exertion of vision. Attention then is to consciousness what the contraction of the pupil is to sight, or, to the eye of the mind what the microscope or telescope is to the bodily eye. It constitutes the better half of all intellectual power."

And *Brodie* adds, quite forcibly: "It is Attention much more than any difference in the abstract power of reasoning, which constitutes the vast difference which exists between minds of different individuals."

Butler gives us this important testimony: "The most important intellectual habit I know of is the habit of attending exclusively to the matter in hand. It is commonly said that genius cannot be infused by education, yet this power of concentrated attention, which belongs as a part of his gift to every great discoverer, is unquestionably capable of almost indefinite augmentation by resolute practice."

And, concluding this review of opinions, and endorsements of that which the Yogis have so much to say, and to which they attach so much importance, let us listen to the words of *Beattie*, who says: "The force wherewith anything strikes the mind, is generally in proportion to the degree of attention bestowed upon it. Moreover, the great art of memory is attention, and inattentive people always have bad memories."

There are two general kinds of Attention. The first is the Attention directed within the mind upon mental objects and concepts. The other is the Attention directed outward upon objects external to ourselves. The same general rules and laws apply to both equally.

Likewise, there may be drawn another distinction and division of attention into two classes, *viz.*, Attention attracted by some impression coming into consciousness without any conscious effort of the Will—this is called Involuntary Attention, for the Attention and Interest is caught by the attractiveness or novelty of the object. Attention directed to some object by an effort of the Will, is called Voluntary Attention. Involuntary Attention is quite common, and requires no special training. In fact, the lower animals, and young children seem to have a greater share of it than do adult men. A great percentage of men and women never get beyond this stage to any marked degree.

On the other hand, Voluntary Attention requires effort, will, and determination—a certain mental training, that is beyond the majority of people, for they will not "take the trouble" to direct their attention in this way. Voluntary Attention is the mark of the student and other thoughtful men. They focus their minds on objects that do not yield immediate interest or pleasure, in order that they may learn and accomplish. The careless person will not thus fasten his Attention, at least not more than a moment or so, for his Involuntary Attention is soon attracted by some passing object of no matter how trifling a nature, and the Voluntary Attention disappears and is forgotten. Voluntary Attention is developed by practice and perseverance, and is well worth the trouble, for nothing in the mental world is accomplished without its use.

The Attention does not readily fasten itself to uninteresting objects, and, unless interest can be created it requires a considerable degree of Voluntary Attention in order that the mind may be fastened upon such an object. And, more than this, even if the ordinary attention is attracted it will soon waver, unless there is some interesting change in the aspect of the object, that will give the attention a fresh hold of interest, or unless some new quality, characteristic or property manifests itself in the object. This fact occurs because the mind mechanism has not been trained to bear prolonged Voluntary Attention, and, in fact, the physical brain is not accustomed to the task, although it may be so trained by patient practice.

It has been noticed by investigators that the Attention may be rested and freshened, either by withdrawing the Voluntary Attention from the object, and allowing the Attention to manifest along Involuntary lines toward passing objects, etc.; or, on the other hand, by directing the Voluntary Attention into a new field of observation—toward some new object. Sometimes one plan will seem to give the best results, and again the other will seem preferable.

We have called your attention to the fact that Interest develops Attention, and holds it fixed, while an uninteresting object or subject requires a much greater effort and application. This fact is apparent to anyone. A common illustration may be found in the matter of reading a book. Nearly everyone will give his undivided attention to some bright, thrilling story, while but few are able to use sufficient Voluntary Attention to master the pages of some scientific work. But, right here, we wish to call your attention to the other side of the case, which is another example of the fact that Truth is composed of paradoxes.

Just as Interest develops Attention, so it is a truth that Attention develops Interest. If one will take the trouble to give a little Voluntary Attention to an object, he will soon find that a little perseverance will bring to light points of Interest in the object. Things before unseen and unsuspected, are quickly brought to light. And many new phases, and aspects of the subject or object are seen, each one of which, in turn, becomes an object of Interest. This is a fact not so generally known, and one that it will be well for you to remember, and to use in practice. *Look* for the interesting features of an uninteresting thing, and they will appear to your view, and before long the uninteresting object will have changed into a thing having many-sided interests.

Voluntary Attention is one of the signs of a developed Will. That is, of a mind that has been well trained by the Will, for the Will is always strong, and it is the mind that has to be trained, not the Will. And on the other hand, one of the best ways to train the mind by the Will, is by practice in Voluntary Attention. So you see how the rule works both ways. Some Western psychologists have even advanced theories that the Voluntary Attention is the *only* power of the Will, and that that power is sufficient, for if the Attention be firmly fixed, and held upon an object the mind will "do the rest." We do not agree with this school of philosophers, but merely mention the fact as an illustration of the importance attributed by psychologists to this matter of Voluntary Attention.

A man of a strongly developed Attention often accomplishes far more than some much brighter man who lacks it. Voluntary Attention and Application is a very good substitute for Genius, and often accomplishes far more in the long run.

Voluntary Attention is the fixing of the mind earnestly and intently upon some particular object, at the same time shutting out from consciousness other objects pressing for entrance. *Hamilton* has defined it as "consciousness voluntarily applied under its law of limitations to some determinate object." The same writer goes on to state that "the greater the number of objects to which our consciousness is simultaneously extended, the smaller is the intensity with which it is able to consider each, and consequently the less vivid and distinct will be the information it contains of the several objects. When our interest in any particular object is excited, and when we wish to obtain all the knowledge concerning it in our power, it behooves us to limit our consideration to that object to the exclusion of others."

The human mind has the power of attending to only one object at a time, although it is able to pass from one object to another with a marvelous degree of speed, so rapidly, in fact, that some have held that it could grasp several things at once. But the best authorities, Eastern and Western, hold to the "single idea" theory as being correct. On this point we may quote a few authorities.

Jouffroy says that "It is established by experience that we cannot give our attention to two different objects at the same time." And *Holland* states that "Two thoughts, however closely related to one another, cannot be presumed to exist at the same time." And *Lewes* has told us that "The nature of our organism prevents our having more than one aspect of an object at each instant presented to consciousness." *Whateley* says: "The best philosophers are agreed that the mind cannot actually attend to more than one thing at a time, but, when it appears to be doing so it is really shifting with prodigious rapidity backward and forward from one to the other."

By giving a concentrated Voluntary Attention to an object, we not only are able to see and think about it with the greatest possible degree of clearness, but the mind has a tendency, under such circumstances, to bring into the field of consciousness all the different ideas associated in our memory with that object or subject, and to build around the object or subject a mass of associated facts and information. And at the same time the Attention given the subject makes more vivid and clear all that we learn about the thing at the time, and, in fact, all that we may afterwards learn about it. It seems to cut a channel, through which knowledge flows.

Attention magnifies and increases the powers of perception, and greatly aids the exercise of the perceptive faculties. By "paying attention" to something seen or heard, one is enabled to observe the details of the thing seen or heard, and where the inattentive mind acquires say three impressions the attentive mind absorbs three times three, or perhaps three times "three times three," or twenty-seven. And, as we have just said, Attention brings into play the powers of association, and gives us the "loose end" of an almost infinite chain of associated facts, stored away in our memory, forming new combinations of facts which we had never grouped together before, and bring out into the field of consciousness all the many scraps of information regarding the thing to which we are giving attention. The proof of this is within the experience of everyone.

Where is the one who does not remember sitting down to some writing, painting, reading, etc., with interest and attention, and finding, much to his surprise, what a flow of facts regarding the matter in hand was passing through his mind. Attention seems to focus all the knowledge of a thing that you possess, and by bringing it to a point enables you to combine, associate, classify, etc., and thus create new knowledge. *Gibbon* tells us that after he gave a brief glance and consideration to a new subject, he suspended further work upon it, and allowed his mind (under concentrated attention) to bring forth all his associated knowledge regarding the subject, after which he renewed the task with increased power and efficiency.

The more one's attention is fixed upon a subject under consideration, the deeper is the impression which the subject leaves upon the mind. And the easier will it be for him to afterwards pursue the same train of thought and work.

Attention is a prerequisite of good memory, and in fact there can be no memory at all unless some degree of attention is given. The degree of memory depends upon the degree of attention and interest. And when it is considered that the work of today is made efficient by the memory of things learned yesterday, the day before yesterday, and so on, it is seen that the degree of attention given today regulates the quality of the work of tomorrow.

Some authorities have described Genius as the result of great powers of attention, or, at least, that the two seem to run together. Some writer has said that "possibly the best definition of genius is the power of concentrating upon someone given subject until its possibilities are exhausted and absorbed." *Simpson* has said that "The power and habit of thinking closely and continuously upon the subject at hand, to the exclusion, for the time, of all other subjects, is one of the principal, if, indeed, not the principal, means of success." *Sir Isaac Newton* has told us his plan of absorbing information and knowledge. He has stated that he would keep the subject under consideration before him continually, and then would wait till the first dawning of perception gradually brightened into a clear light, little by little. A mental sunrise, in fact.

That sage observer, *Dr. Abercrombie*, has written that he considered that he knew of no more important rule for rising to eminence in any profession or occupation than the Ability to do one thing at a time, avoiding all distracting and diverting objects or subjects, and keeping the leading matter continually before the mind. And others have added that such a course will enable one to observe relations between the subject and other things that will not be apparent to the careless observer or student.

The degree of Attention cultivated by a man is the degree of his capacity for intellectual work. As we have said, the "great" men of all walks of life have developed this faculty to a wonderful degree, and many of them seem to get results "intuitively," whereas, in truth, they obtain them by reason of their concentrated power of Attention, which enables them to see right into the center of a subject or proposition—and all around it, back and front, and all sides, in a space of time incredible to the man who has not cultivated this mighty power. Men who have devoted much attention to some special line of work or research, are able to act almost as if they possessed "second sight," providing the subject is within their favorite field of endeavor. Attention quickens every one of the faculties—the reasoning faculties—the senses—the deriding qualities—the analytical faculties, and so on, each being given a "fine edge" by their use under a concentrated Attention.

And, on the other hand, there is no surer indication of a weak mind than the deficiency in Attention. This weakness may arise from illness or physical weakness reacting upon the brain, in which case the trouble is but temporary. Or it may arise from a lack of mental development. Imbeciles and idiots have little or no Attention. The great French psychologist, *Luys*, speaking of this fact, says "Imbeciles and idiots see badly, hear badly, feel badly, and their sensorium is, in consequence, in a similar condition of sensitive poverty. Its impressionability for the things of the external world is at a minimum, its sensibility weak, and consequently, it is difficult to provoke the physiological condition necessary for the absorption of the external impression."

In old age the Attention is the first faculty to show signs of decay. Some authorities have held that the Memory was the first faculty to be affected by the approach of old age, but this is incorrect, for it is a matter of common experience that the aged manifest a wonderfully clear memory of events occurring in the far past. The reason that their memory of recent events is so poor is because their failing powers of Attention has prevented them from receiving strong, clear mental impressions, and as is the impression so is the memory. Their early impressions having been clear and strong, are easily recalled, while their later ones, being weak, are recalled with difficulty. If the Memory were at fault, it would be difficult for them to recall any impression, recent or far distant in time.

But we must stop quoting examples and authorities, and urging upon you the importance of the faculty of Attention. If you do not now realize it, it is because you have not given the subject the Attention that you should have exercised, and further repetition would not remedy matters.

Admitting the importance of Attention, from the psychological point of view, not to speak of the occult side of the subject, is it not a matter of importance for you to start in to cultivate that faculty? We think so. And the only way to cultivate any mental or physical part or faculty is to Exercise it. Exercise "uses up" a muscle, or mental faculty, but the organism makes haste to rush to the scene additional material—cell-stuff, nerve force, etc., to repair the waste, and it always sends a little more than is needed. And this "little more," continually accruing and increasing, is what increases the muscles and brain centers. And improved and strengthened brain centers give the mind better instruments with which to work.

One of the first things to do in the cultivation of Attention is to learn to think of, and do, one thing at a time. Acquiring the "knack" or habit of attending closely to the things before us, and then passing on to the next and treating it in the same way, is most conducive to success, and its practice is the best exercise for the cultivation of the faculty of Attention. And on the contrary, there is nothing more harmful from the point of view of successful performance—and nothing that will do more to destroy the power of giving Attention—than the habit of trying to do one thing while thinking of another. The thinking part of the mind, and the acting part should work together, not in opposition.

Dr. Beattie, speaking of this subject, tells us "It is a matter of no small importance that we acquire the habit of doing only one thing at a time; by which I mean that while attending to any one object, our thoughts ought not to wander to another." And *Granville* adds, "A frequent cause of failure in the faculty of Attention is striving to think of more than one thing at a time." And *Kay* quotes, approvingly, a writer who says: "She did things easily, because she attended to them in the doing. When she made bread, she thought of the bread, and not of the fashion of her next dress, or of her partner at the last dance." *Lord Chesterfield said,* "There is time enough for everything in the course of the day, if you do but one thing at a time; but there is not time enough in the year if you try to do two things at a time."

To attain the best results, one should practice concentrating upon the task before him, shutting out, so far as possible, every other idea or thought. One should even forget self—personality—in such cases, as there is nothing more destructive of good thinking than to allow morbid self-consciousness to intrude. One does best when he "forgets himself" in his work, and sinks his personality in the creative work. The "earnest" man or woman is the one who sinks personality in the desired result, or performance of the task undertaken. The actor, or preacher, or orator, or writer, must lose sight of himself to get the best results. Keep the Attention fixed on the thing before you, and let the self-take care of itself.

In connection with the above, we may relate an anecdote of *Whateley* that may be interesting in connection with the consideration of this subject of "losing one's self" in the task. He was asked for a recipe for "bashfulness," and replied that the person was bashful simply because he was thinking of himself and the impression he was making. His recipe was that the young man should think of others—of the pleasure he could give them—and in that way he would forget all about himself. The prescription is said to have affected the cure. The same authority has written, "Let both the extemporary speaker, and the reader of his own compositions, study to avoid as far as possible all thoughts of self, earnestly fixing the mind on the matter of what is delivered; and they will feel less that embarrassment which arises from the thought of what opinion the hearers will form of them."

The same writer, *Whateley*, seems to have made quite a study of Attention and has given us some interesting information on its details. The following may be read with interest, and if properly understood may be employed to advantage. He says, "It is a fact, and a very curious one. that many people find that they can best attend to any serious matter when they are occupied with something else which requires a little, and but a little, attention, such as working with the needle, cutting open paper leaves, or, for want of some such employment, fiddling anyhow with the fingers."

He does not give the reason for this, and at first sight it might seem like a contradiction of the "one thing at a time" idea. But a closer examination will show us that the minor work (the cutting leaves, etc.) is in the nature of an involuntary or automatic movement, inasmuch as it requires little or no voluntary attention, and seems to "do itself." It does not take off the Attention from the main subject, but perhaps acts to catch the "waste Attention" that often tries to divide the Attention from some voluntary act to another.

The habit mind may be doing one thing, while the Attention is fixed on another. For instance, one may be writing with his attention firmly fixed upon the thought he wishes to express, while at the time his hand is doing the writing, apparently with no attention being given it. But, let a boy, or person unaccustomed to writing, try to express his thoughts in this way, and you will find that he is hampered in the flow of his thoughts by the fact that he has to give much attention to the mechanical act of writing. In the same way, the beginner on the typewriter finds it difficult to compose to the machine, while the experienced typist finds the mechanical movements no hindrance whatever to the flow of thought and focusing of Attention; in fact, many find that they can compose much better while using the typewriter than they can by dictating to a stenographer. We think you will see the principle.

And now for a little Mental Drill in Attention, that you may be started on the road to cultivate this important faculty.

MENTAL DRILL IN ATTENTION

Exercise I. Begin by taking some familiar object and placing it before you, try to get as many impressions regarding it as is possible for you. Study its shape, its color, its size, and the thousand and one little peculiarities about it that present themselves to your attention. In doing this, reduce the thing to its simplest parts—analyze it as far as is possible—dissect it, mentally, and study its parts in detail. The simpler and smaller the part to be considered, the more clearly will the impression be received, and the more vividly will it be recalled. Reduce the thing to the smallest possible proportions, and then examine each portion, and mastering that, then pass on to the next part, and so on, until you have covered the entire field. Then, when you have exhausted the object, take a pencil and paper and put down as nearly as possible all the things or details of the object examined. When you have done this, compare the written description with the object itself, and see how many things you have failed to note.

The next day take up the same object, and after re-examining it, write down the details and you will find that you will have stored away a greater number of impressions regarding it, and, moreover, you will have discovered many new details during your second examination. This exercise strengthens the memory as well as the Attention, for the two are closely connected, the memory depending largely upon the clearness and strength of the impressions received, while the impressions depend upon the amount of attention given to the thing observed. Do not tire yourself with this exercise, for a tired Attention is a poor Attention. Better try it by degrees, increasing the task a little each time you try it. Make a game of it if you like, and you will find it quite interesting to notice the steady but gradual improvement.

It will be interesting to practice this in connection with some friend, varying the exercise by both examining the object, and writing down their impressions, separately, and then comparing results. This adds interest to the task, and you will be surprised to see how rapidly both of you increase in your powers of observation, which powers, of course, result from Attention.

Exercise II. This exercise is but a variation of the first one. It consists in entering a room, and taking a hasty glance around, and then walking out, and afterward writing down the number of things that you have observed, with a description of each. You will be surprised to observe how many things you have missed at first sight, and how you will improve in observation by a little practice. This exercise, also, may be improved by the assistance of a friend, as related in our last exercise. It is astonishing how many details one may observe and remember, after a little practice. It is related of Houdin, the French conjurer, that he improved and developed his faculty of Attention and Memory by playing this game with a young relative. They would pass by a shop window, taking a hasty, attentive glance at its contents. Then they would go around the corner and compare notes.

At first, they could remember only a few prominent articles—that is, their Attention could grasp only a few. But as they developed by practice, they found that they could observe and remember a vast number of things and objects in the window. And, at last, it is related that Houdin could pass rapidly before any large shop window, bestowing upon it but one hasty glance, and then tell the names of, and closely describe, nearly every object in plain sight in the window. The feat was accomplished by the fact that the cultivated Attention enabled Houdin to fasten upon his mind a vivid mental image of the window and its contents, and then he was able to describe the articles one by one from the picture in his mind.

Houdin taught his son to develop Attention by a simple exercise which may be interesting and of value to you. He would lay down a domino before the boy—a five-four, for example. He would require the boy to tell him the combined number at once, without allowing him to stop to count the spots, one by one. "Nine" the boy would answer after a moment's hesitation. Then another domino, a three-four, would be added. "That makes sixteen," cried the boy.

Two dominoes at a time was the second day's task. The next day, three was the standard. The next day, four, and so on, until the boy was able to handle twelve dominoes—that is to say, give instantaneously the total number of spots on twelve dominoes, after a single glance. This was Attention, in earnest, and shows what practice will do to develop a faculty. The result was shown by the wonderful powers of observation, memory and attention, together with instantaneous mental action, that the boy developed. Not only was he able to add dominoes instantaneously, but he had powers of observation, etc., that seemed little short of miraculous. And yet it is related that he had poor attention, and deficient memory to begin with.

If this seems incredible, let us remember how old whist players note and remember every card in the pack, and can tell whether they have been played or not, and all the circumstances attending upon them. The same is true of chess players, who observe every move and can relate the whole game in detail long after it has been played. And remember, also, how one woman may pass another woman on the street, and without seeming to give her more than a careless glance, may be able to relate in detail every feature of the other woman's apparel, including its color, texture, style of fashioning, probable price of the material, etc., etc.

And a mere man would have noticed scarcely anything about it—because he would not have given it any attention. But how soon would that man learn to equal his sister in attention and observation of women's wearing apparel, if his business success depended upon it, or if his speculative instinct was called into play by a wager with some friend as to who could remember the most about a woman's clothing, seen in a passing glance? You see it is all a matter of Interest and Attention.

But we forget that the Attention may be developed and cultivated, and we complain that we "cannot remember things," or that we do not seem to be able to "take notice." A little practice will do wonders in this direction.

Now, while the above exercises will develop your memory and powers of observation, still that is not the main reason that we have given them to you. We have an ulterior object, that will appear in time. We aim to develop your Will-power, and we know that Attention stands at the gate of Will-power. In order to be able to use your Will, you must be able to focus the Attention forcibly and distinctly. And these childish exercises will help you to develop the mental muscles of the Attention. If you could but realize the childish games the young Yogi students are required to play, in order to develop the mental faculties, you would change your minds about the Yogi Adepts whom you have been thinking about as mere dreamers, far removed from the practical.

These men, and their students, are intensely practical. They have gained the mastery of the Mind, and its faculties, and are able to use them as sharp-edged tools, while the untrained man finds that he has but a dull, unsharpened blade that will do nothing but hack and hew roughly, instead of being able to produce the finished product.

The Yogi believes in giving the "I" good tools with which to work, and he spends much time in tempering and sharpening these tools. Oh, no, the Yogi are not idle dreamers. Their grasp of "practical things" would surprise many a practical, matter-of-fact Western business man, if he could but observe it.

And so, we ask you to practice "observing things." The two exercises we have given are but indications of the general line. We could give you thousands, but you can prepare them yourselves as well as could we. The little Hindu boy is taught Attention by being asked to note and remember the number, color, character and other details of a number of colored stones, jewelry, etc., shown for an instant in an open palm, the hand being closed the moment after.

He is taught to note and describe passing travelers, and their equipages—houses he sees on his journeys—and thousands of other everyday objects. The results are almost marvelous. In this way he is prepared as a *chela* or student, and he brings to his *guru* or teacher a brain well developed—a mind thoroughly trained to obey the Will of the "I"—and with faculties quickened to perceive instantly that which others would fail to see in a fortnight. It is true that he does not turn these faculties to "business" or other so-called "practical" pursuits, but prefers to devote them to abstract studies and pursuits outside of that which the Western man considers to be the end and aim of life. But remember that the two civilizations are quite different—following different ideals—having different economic conditions—living in different worlds, as it were. But that is all a matter of taste and ideals—the faculty for the "practical life" of the West is possessed by the *chela*, if he saw fit to use it. But all Hindu youths are not *chelas*, remember—nor are all Western youths "captains of industry," or Edisons.

MANTRAM (AFFIRMATION)

I am using my Attention to develop my mental faculties, so as to give the "I" a perfect instrument with which to work. The mind is *My* instrument and I am bringing it to a state of capacity for perfect work.

MANTRAM (OR AFFIRMATION)

There is but One Life—One Life Underlying. This Life is manifesting through ME, and through every other shape, form, and thing. I am resting on the bosom of the Great Ocean of Life, and it is supporting me, and will carry me safely, though the waves rise and fall—though the storms rage and the tempests roar. I am safe on the Ocean of Life, and rejoice as I feel the sway of its motion. Nothing can harm me—though changes may come and go, I am Safe. I am One with the All Life, and its Power, Knowledge, and Peace are behind, underneath, and within Me. O! One Life! express Thyself through me—carry me now on the crest of the wave, now deep down in the trough of the ocean—supported always by Thee—all is good to me, as I feel Thy life moving in and through me. I am Alive, through thy life, and I open myself to thy full manifestation and inflow.

THE SIXTH LESSON

CULTIVATION OF PERCEPTION.

Man gains his knowledge of the outside world through his senses. And, consequently, many of us are in the habit of thinking of these senses as if *they* did the sensing, instead of being merely carriers of the vibrations coming from the outside world, which are then presented to the Mind for examination. We shall speak of this at greater length a little later on in this lesson. Just now we wish to impress upon you the fact that it is the Mind that perceives, not the senses. And, consequently, a development of Perception is really a development of the Mind.

The Yogis put their students through a very arduous course of practice and exercises designed to develop their powers of perception. To many this would appear to be merely a development of the Senses, which might appear odd in view of the fact that the Yogis are constantly preaching the folly of being governed and ruled by the senses. But there is nothing paradoxical about all this, for the Yogis, while preaching the folly of sense life, and manifesting the teaching in their lives, nevertheless believe in any and all exercises calculated to "sharpen" the Mind, and develop it to a keen state and condition.

They see a great difference between having a sharpened perception, on the one hand, and being a slave to the senses on the other. For instance, what would be thought of a man who objected to acquiring a keen eyesight, for fear it would lead him away from higher things, by reason of his becoming attached to the beautiful things he might see. To realize the folly of this idea, one may look at its logical conclusion, which would be that one would then be much better off if all their senses were destroyed. The absurdity, not to say wickedness, of such an idea will be apparent to everyone, after a minute's consideration.

The secret of the Yogi theory and teachings regarding the development of the Mental powers, lies in the word "*Mastery*." The Yoga student accomplishes and attains this mastery in two ways. The first way is by subordinating all the feelings, sense-impressions, etc., to the Mastery of the "I," or Will, the Mastery being obtained in this way by the assertion of the dominancy of the "I" over the faculties and emotions, etc. The second step, or way, lies in the Yogi, once having asserted the mastery, beginning to develop and perfect the Mental instrument, so as to get better work and returns from it. In this way he increases his kingdom and is Master over a much larger territory.

In order for one to gain knowledge, it is necessary to use to the best advantage the mental instruments and tools that he finds at his disposal. And again, one must develop and improve such tools—put a keen edge upon them, etc. Not only does one gain a great benefit from a development of the faculties of perception, but he also acquires an additional benefit from the training of the whole mind arising from the mental discipline and training resulting from the former exercises, etc. In our previous lessons we have pointed out some of the means by which these faculties might be greatly improved, and their efficiency increased. In this lesson we shall point out certain directions in which the Perceptive faculties may be trained.

We trust that the simplicity of the idea may not cause any of our students to lose interest in the work. If they only knew just what such development would lead to, they would gladly follow our suggestions in the matter. Every one of the ideas and exercises given by us are intended to lead up to the strengthening of the Mind, and the attainment of powers and the unfoldment of faculties. There is no royal road to Raja Yoga, but the student will be well repaid for the work of climbing the hill of Attainment.

In view of the above, let us examine the question of The Senses. Through the doors of the senses Man receives all his information regarding the outside world. If he keeps these doors but half open, or crowded up with obstacles and rubbish, he may expect to receive but few messages from outside. But if he keeps his doorways clear, and clean, he will obtain the best that is passing his way.

If one were born without sense-organs—no matter how good a Mind he might have—he would be compelled to live his life in a dreamy plant-life stage of existence, with little or no consciousness. The Mind would be like a seed in the earth, that for some reason was prevented from growing.

One may object that the highest ideas do not come to us through the senses, but the reply is that the things obtained through the senses are the "raw material" upon which the mind works, and fashions the beautiful things that it is able to produce in its highest stages. Just as is the body dependent for growth upon the nourishment taken into it, so is the mind dependent for growth upon the impressions received from the Universe—and these impressions come largely through the senses. It may be objected to that we know many things that we have not received through our senses. But, does the objector include the impressions that came through his senses in some previous existence, and which have been impressed upon his instinctive mind, or soul-memory? It is true that there are higher senses than those usually recognized, but Nature insists upon one learning the lessons of the lower grades before attempting those of the higher.

Do not forget that all that we know we have "worked for." There is nothing that comes to the idler, or shirker. What we know is merely the result of "stored-up accumulations of previous experience," as Lewes has so well said.

So, it will be seen that the Yogi idea that one should develop all parts of the Mind is strictly correct, if one will take the trouble to examine into the matter. A man sees and knows but very little of what is going on about him. His limitations are great. His powers of vision report only a few vibrations of light, while below and above the scale lie an infinity of vibrations unknown to him. The same is true of the powers of hearing, for only a comparatively small portion of the sound-waves reach the Mind of Man—even some of the animals hear more than he does.

If a man had only one sense, he would obtain but a one-sense idea of the outside world. If another sense is added his knowledge is doubled. And so on. The best proof of the relation between increased sense perception and development is had in the study of the evolution of animal forms. In the early stages of life, the organism has only the sense of feeling—and very dim at that—and a faint sense of taste. Then developed smell, hearing and sight, each marking a distinct advance in the scale of life, for a new world has been opened out to the advancing forms of life. And, when man develops new senses—and this is before the race—he will be a much wiser and greater being.

Carpenter, many years ago, voiced a thought that will be familiar to those who are acquainted with the Yogi teachings regarding the unfoldment of new senses. He said: "It does not seem at all improbable that there are properties of matter of which none of our senses can take immediate cognizance, and which other beings might be formed to perceive in the same manner as we are sensible to light, sound, etc."

And Isaac Taylor said: "It may be that within the field observed by the visible and ponderable universe there is existing and moving another element fraught with another species of life—corporeal, indeed, and various in its orders, but not open to cognizance of those who are confined to the conditions of animal organization. Is it to be thought that the eye of man is the measure of the Creator's power? - and that He created nothing but that which he has exposed to our present senses? The contrary seems much more than barely possible; ought we not to think it almost certain?"

Another writer. Prof. Masson, has said: "If a new sense or two were added to the present normal number, in man, that which is now the phenomenal world for all of us might, for all that we know, burst into something amazingly different and wider, in consequence of the additional revelations of these new senses."

But not only is this true, but Man may increase his powers of knowledge and experience if he will but develop the senses he has to a higher degree of efficiency, instead of allowing them to remain comparatively atrophied. And toward this end, this lesson is written.

The Mind obtains its impressions of objects of the outside world by means of the brain and sense organs. The sensory organs are the instruments of the Mind, as is also the brain and the entire nervous system. By means of the nerves, and the brain, the Mind makes use of the sensory organs in order that it may obtain information regarding external objects.

The senses are usually said to consist of five different forms, *viz.*, sight, hearing, smell, touch, and taste.

The Yogis teach that there are higher senses, undeveloped, or comparatively so, in the majority of the race, but toward the unfoldment of which the race is tending. But we shall not touch upon these latent senses in this lesson, as they belong to another phase of the subject. In addition to the five senses above enumerated, some physiologists and psychologists have held that there were several others in evidence. For instance, the sense by which the inner organs revealed their presence and condition, the muscular system reports to the mind through some sense that is not that of "touch," although closely allied to it. And the feelings of hunger, thirst, etc., seem to come to us through an unnamed sense.

Bernstein has distinguished between the five senses and the one just referred to as follows: "The characteristic distinction between these common sensations and the sensations of the senses is that by the latter we gain knowledge of the occurrences and objects which belong to the external world (and which sensations we refer to external objects), whilst by the former we only feel conditions of our own body."

A sensation is the internal, mental conception, resulting from an external object or fact exciting the sense organs and nerves, and the brain, thus making the mind "aware" of the external object or fact. As Bain has said, it is the "mental impression, feeling, or conscious state, resulting from the action of external things on some part of the body, called on that account, sensitive."

Each channel of sense impressions has an organ, or organs, peculiarly adapted for the excitation of its substance by the particular kind of vibrations through which it receives impressions. The eye is most cunningly and carefully designed to receive the light-waves; and sound-waves produce no effect upon it. And, likewise, the delicate mechanism of the ear responds only to sound-waves; light-waves failing to register upon it. Each set of sensations is entirely different, and the organs and nerves designed to register each particular set are peculiarly adapted to their own special work. The organs of sense, including their special nervous systems, may be compared to a delicate instrument that the mind has fashioned for itself, that it may investigate, examine and obtain reports from the outside world.

We have become so accustomed to the workings of the senses that we take them as a "matter of course," and fail to recognize them as the delicate and wonderful instruments that they are—designed and perfected by the mind for its own use. If we will think of the soul as designing, manufacturing and using these instruments, we may begin to understand their true relations to our lives, and, accordingly treat them with more respect and consideration.

We are in the habit of thinking that we are aware of all the sensations received by our mind. But this is very far from being correct. The unconscious regions of the mind are incomparably larger than the small conscious area that we generally think of when we say "my mind."

In future lessons we shall proceed to consider this wonderful area, and examine what is to be found there. Taine has well said, "There is going on within us a subterranean process of infinite extent; its products alone are known to us, and are only known to us in the mass. As to elements, and their elements, consciousness does not attain to them. They are to sensations what secondary molecules and primitive molecules are to bodies. We get a glance here and there at obscure and infinite worlds extending beneath our distinct sensations. These are compounds and wholes. For their elements to be perceptible to consciousness, it is necessary for them to be added together, and so to acquire a certain bulk and to occupy a certain time, for if the group does not attain this bulk, and does not last this time, we observe no changes in our state. Nevertheless, though it escapes us, there is one."

But we must postpone our consideration of this more than interesting phase of the subject, until some future lesson, when we shall take a trip into the regions of Mind, under and above Consciousness. And a most wonderful trip many of us will find it, too.

For the present, we must pay our attention to the channels by which the material for knowledge and thought enter our minds. For these sense impressions, coming to us from without, are indeed "material" upon which the mind works in order to manufacture the product called "Thought."

This material we obtain through the channels of the senses, and then store in that wonderful storehouse, the Memory, from whence we bring out material from time to time, which we proceed to weave into the fabric of Thought. The skill of the worker depends upon his training, and his ability to select and combine the proper materials. And the acquiring of good materials to be stored up is an important part of the work.

A mind without stored-up material of impressions and experiences would be like a factory without material. The machinery would have nothing upon which to work, and the shop would be idle. As Helmholtz has said, "Apprehension by the senses supplies directly or indirectly, the material of all human knowledge, or at least the stimulus necessary to develop every inborn faculty of the mind." And Herbert Spencer, has this to say of this phase of the subject, "It is almost a truism to say that in proportion to the numerousness of the objects that can be distinguished, and in proportion to the variety of coexistences and sequences that can be severally responded to, must be the number and rapidity and variety of the changes within the organism—must be the amount of vitality."

A little reflection upon this subject will show us that the greater degree of exercise and training given the senses, the greater the degree of mental power and capability. As we store our mental storehouse with the materials to be manufactured into thought, so is the quality and quantity of the fabric produced.

It therefore behooves us to awaken from our "lazy" condition of mind, and to proceed to develop our organs of sense, and their attendant mechanism, as by doing so we increase our capacity for thought and knowledge.

Before passing to the exercises, however, it may be well to give a hasty passing glance at the several senses, and their peculiarities.

The sense of Touch is the simplest and primal sense. Long before the lower forms of life had developed the higher senses, they had evidenced the sense of Touch or Feeling. Without this sense they would have been unable to have found their food, or to receive and respond to outside impressions. In the early forms of life, it was exercised equally by all parts of the body, although in the higher forms this sense has become somewhat localized, as certain parts of the body are far more sensitive than are others. The skin is the seat of the sense of Touch, and its nerves are distributed over the entire area of the skin. The hand, and particularly the fingers, and their tips, are the principal organs of this sense.

The acuteness of Touch varies materially in different parts of the body. Experiments have shown that a pair of compasses would register impressions as a very slight distance apart when applied to the tip of the tongue. The distance at which the two points could be distinguished from one point, on the tip of the tongue, was called "one line." Using this "line" as a standard, it was found that the palmar surface of the third finger registered 2 lines; the surface of the lips 4 lines, and the skin of the back, and on the middle of the arm or thigh, as high as 60 lines The degree of sensitiveness to Touch varies greatly with different individuals, some having a very fine sense of touch in their fingers, while others manifested a very much lower degree.

In the same way, there is a great difference in the response of the fingers to weight—a great difference in the ability to distinguish the difference of the weight of objects. It has been found that some people can distinguish differences in weight down to very small fractions of an ounce. Fine distinctions in the differences in temperature have also been noticed.

The sense of touch, and its development has meant much for Man. It is the one sense in which Man surpasses the animals in the matter of degree and acuteness. The animal may have a keener smell, taste, hearing and sight, but its sense of Touch is far beneath that of Man. Anaxagoras is quoted as saying that "if the animals had hands and fingers, they would be like men."

In developing the sense of Touch, the student must remember that Attention is the key to success. The greater the amount of Attention the greater the degree of development possible in the case of any sense. When the Attention is concentrated upon any particular sense, the latter becomes quickened and more acute, and repeated exercise, under the stimulus of Attention, will work wonders in the case of any particular sense. And on the other hand, the sense of touch may be almost, or completely inhibited, by firmly fixing the Attention upon something else. As an extreme proof of this latter fact, the student is asked to remember the fact that men have been known to suffer excruciating torture, apparently without feeling, owing to the mind being intently riveted upon some idea or thought.

As Wyld has said, "The martyr borne above sensuous impressions, is not only able to endure tortures, but is able to endure and quench them. The pinching and cutting of the flesh only added energy to the death song of the American Indian, and even the slave under the lash is sustained by the indignant sense of his wrongs."

In the cases of persons engaged in occupations requiring a fine degree of Touch, the development is marvelous. The engraver passes his hand over the plate, and is able to distinguish the slightest imperfection. And the handler of cloth and fabrics is able to distinguish the finest differences, simply by the sense of touch. Wool sorters also exercise a wonderfully high degree of fineness of touch. And the blind are able to make up for the loss of sight by their greatly increased sense of Touch, cases being recorded where the blind have been able to distinguish *color* by the different "feel" of the material.

The sense of Taste is closely allied to that of Touch—in fact some authorities have considered Taste as a very highly developed sense of Touch in certain surfaces of the body, the tongue notably. It will be remembered that the tongue has the finest sense of Touch, and it also has the sense of Taste developed to perfection. In Taste and Touch the object must be brought in direct contact with the organ of sense, which is not the case in Smell, Hearing, or Sight. And, be it remembered, that the latter senses have special nerves, while Taste is compelled to fall back upon the ordinary nerves of Touch. It is true that Taste is confined to a very small part of the surface of the body, while Touch is general. But this only indicates a special development of the special area. The sense of Taste also depends to a great extent upon the presence of fluids, and only substances that are soluble make their presence known through the organs and sense of Taste.

Physiologists report that the sense of Taste in some persons is so acute that one part of strychnine in one million parts of water has been distinguished. There are certain occupations, such as that of wine-tasters, tea-tasters, etc., the followers of which manifest a degree of fineness of Taste almost incredible.

The sense of Smell is closely connected with the sense of Taste, and often acts in connection therewith, as the tiny particles of the substance in the mouth arise to the organs of Smell, by means of the opening or means of communication situated in the back part of the mouth. Besides which the nose usually detects the odor of substances before they enter the mouth. The sense of Smell operates by reason of the tiny particles or the object being carried to the mucous membrane of the interior of the nose, by means of the air. The membrane, being moist, seizes and holds these particles for a moment, and the fine nervous organism reports differences and qualities and the Mind is thus informed of the nature of the object.

The sense of Smell is very highly developed among animals, who are compelled to rely upon it to a considerable extent. And many occupations among men require the development of this sense, for instance, the tobacconist, the wine dealer, the perfumers, the chemist, etc. It is related that in the cases of certain blind people, it has been observed that they could distinguish persons in this manner.

The sense of Hearing is a more complex one than in the case of Taste, Touch and Smell. In the latter three the objects to be sensed must be brought in close contact with the sense-organs, while in Hearing the object may be far removed, the impressions being carried by the vibrations of the air, which are caught up and reported upon by the nervous organism of the sense of Hearing. The internal mechanism of the ear is most wonderfully intricate and complex, and excites to wonder the person examining it. It cannot be described here for want of space, but the student is advised to inquire into it if he has access to any library containing books on the subject. It is a wonderful illustration of the work of the mind in building up for itself instruments with which to work—to acquire knowledge.

The ear records vibrations in the air from 20 or 32 per second, the rate of the lowest audible note, to those of 38,000 per second, the rate of the highest audible note. There is a great difference in individuals in regard to the fineness of the sense of Hearing. But all may develop this sense by the application of Attention. The animals and savages have wonderfully acute senses of Hearing developed only along the lines of distinctness, however—on the other hand musicians have developed the sense along different lines.

The sense of Sight is generally conceded to be the highest and most complex of all the senses of Man. It deals with a far larger number of objects—at longer distances—and gives a far greater variety of reports to the mind than any of its associate senses. It is the sense of Touch magnified many times. As Wilson says of it, "Our sight may be considered as a more delicate and diffusive kind of touch that spreads itself over an infinite number of bodies; comprehends the largest figures, and brings into our reach some of the most remote parts of the universe."

The sense of Sight receives its impressions from the outside world by means of waves that travel from body to body—from sun to earth, and from lamp to eye. These waves of light arise from vibrations in substance, of an almost incredible degree of rapidity. The lowest light vibration is about 450,000,000,000,000 per second, while the highest is about 750,000,000,000,000 per second. These figures deal only with the vibrations recognizable by the eye as light. Above and below these figures of the scale are countless other degrees invisible to the eye, although some of them may be recorded by instruments. The different sensations of color, depend upon the rate of the vibrations, red being the limit of the lowest, and violet the limit of the highest visible vibrations—orange, yellow, green, blue, and indigo being the intermediate rates or colors.

The cultivation of the sense of Sight, under the aid of Attention is most important to ail persons. By being able to clearly see and distinguish the parts of an object, a degree of knowledge regarding it is obtained that one may not acquire without the said exercise of the faculty. We have spoken of this under the subject of Attention, in a previous lesson, to which lesson we again refer the student. The fixing of the eye upon an object has the power of concentrating the thoughts and preventing them from wandering. The eye has other properties and qualities that will be dwelt upon in future lessons. It has other uses than seeing. The influence of the eye is a marvelous thing, and may be cultivated and developed.

We trust that what we have said will bring the student to a realization of the importance of developing the powers of Perception. The senses have been developed by the mind during a long period of evolution and effort that surely would not have been given unless the object in view was worth it all. The "I" insists upon obtaining knowledge of the Universe, and much of this knowledge may be obtained only through the senses. The Yogi student must be "wide awake" and possessed of developed senses and powers of Perception. The senses of Sight and Hearing, the two latest in the scale of Evolutionary growth and unfoldment, must receive a particular degree of attention. The student must make himself "aware" of what is going on about and around him, so that he may "catch" the best vibrations.

It would surprise many Westerners if they could come in contact with a highly developed Yogi, and witness the marvelously finely developed senses he possesses. He is able to distinguish the finest differences in things, and his mind is so trained that, in thought, he may draw conclusions from what he has perceived, in a manner that seems almost "second-sight" to the uninitiated. *In fact, a certain degree of second-sight is possible to one who develops his sense of Sight, under the urge of Attention.* A new world is opened out to such a person. One must learn to master the senses, not only in the direction of being independent of and superior to their urgings, but also in the matter of developing them to a high degree. The development of the physical senses, also has much to do with the development of the "Astral Senses," of which we have spoken in our "Fourteen Lessons," and of which we may have more to say in the present series. The idea of *Raja Yoga* is to render the student the possessor of a highly developed Mind, with highly developed instruments with which the mind may work.

In our future lessons we shall give the student many illustrations, directions, and exercises calculated to develop the different faculties of the mind—not only the ordinary faculties of everyday use, but others hidden behind these familiar faculties and senses. Commencing with the next lesson, we shall present a system of exercises, drills, etc., the purpose of which will be the above-mentioned development of the faculties of the Mind.

In this lesson we shall not attempt to give specific exercises, but will content ourselves with calling the attention of the student to a few general rules underlying the development of Perception.

GENERAL RULES OF PERCEPTION

The first thing to remember in acquiring the art of Perception is that one should not attempt to perceive the whole of a complex thing or object at the same time, or at once. One should consider the object in detail, and then, by grouping the details, he will find that he has considered the whole. Let us take the face of a person as a familiar object. If one tries to perceive a face as a whole, he will find that he will meet with a certain degree of failure, the impression being indistinct and cloudy, it following, also, that the memory of that face will correspond with the original perception.

But let the observer consider the face in detail, first the eyes, then the nose, then the mouth, then the chin, then the hair, then the outline of the face, the complexion, etc., and he will find that he will have acquired a clear and distinct impression or perception of the whole face.

The same rule may be applied to any subject or object. Let us take another familiar illustration. You wish to observe a building. If you simply get a general perception of the building as a whole, you will be able to remember very little about it, except its general outlines, shape, size, color, etc. And a description will prove to be very disappointing. But if you have noted, *in detail*, the material used, the shape of the doors, chimney, roof, porches, decorations, trimmings, ornamentation, size and number of the window-panes etc., etc., the shape and angles of the roof, etc., you will have an *intelligent* idea of the building, in the place of a mere general outline or impression of such as might be acquired by an animal in passing.

We will conclude this lesson with an anecdote of the methods of that famous naturalist Agassiz, in his training of his pupils. His pupils became renowned for their close powers of observation and perception, and their consequent ability to "think" about the things they had seen. Many of them rose to eminent positions, and claimed that this was largely by reason of their careful training.

The tale runs that a new student presented himself to Agassiz one day, asking to be set to work. The naturalist took a fish from a jar in which it had been preserved, and laying it before the young student bade him observe it carefully, and be ready to report upon what he had noticed about the fish. The student was then left alone with the fish. There was nothing especially interesting about that fish—it was like many other fishes that he had seen before. He noticed that it had fins and scales, and a mouth and eyes, yes, and a tail. In a half hour he felt certain that he had observed all about that fish that there was to be perceived. But the naturalist remained away.

The time rolled on, and the youth, having nothing else to do, began to grow restless and weary. He started out to hunt up the teacher, but he failed to find him, and so had to return and gaze again at that wearisome fish. Several hours had passed, and he knew but little more about the fish than he did in the first place.

He went out to lunch and when he returned it was still a case of watching the fish. He felt disgusted and discouraged, and wished he had never come to Agassiz, whom, it seemed, was a stupid old man after all, one away behind the times. Then, in order to kill time, he began to count the scales. This completed he counted the spines of the fins. Then he began to draw a picture of the fish. In drawing the picture, he noticed that the fish had no eyelids. He thus made the discovery that as his teacher had expressed it often, in lectures, "a pencil is the best of eyes." Shortly after the teacher returned, and after ascertaining what the youth had observed, he left rather disappointed, telling the boy to keep on looking and maybe he would see something.

This put the boy on his mettle, and he began to work with his pencil, putting down little details that had escaped him before, but which now seemed very plain to him. He began to catch the secret of observation. Little by little he brought to light new objects of interest about the fish. But this did not suffice his teacher, who kept him at work on the same fish for three whole days. At the end of that time the student really knew something about the fish, and, better than all, had acquired the "knack" and habit of careful observation and perception in detail.

Years after, the student, then attained to eminence, is reported as saying: "That was the best zoological lesson I ever had—a lesson whose influence has extended to the details of every subsequent study; a legacy that the professor left to me, as he left to many others, of inestimable value, which we could not buy, and with which we cannot part."

Apart from the value to the student of the particular information obtained, was the quickening of the perceptive faculties that enabled him to observe the important points in a subject or object, and, consequently to deduce important information from that which was observed. The Mind is hungry for knowledge, and it has by years of weary evolution and effort built up a series of sense systems in order to yield it that knowledge and it is still building. The men and women in the world who have arrived at the point of success have availed themselves of these wonderful channels of information, and by directing them under the guidance of Will and Attention, have attained wonderful results. These things are of importance, and we beg of our students not to pass by this portion of the subject as uninteresting.

Cultivate a spirit of wide-awareness and perception, and the "knowing" that will come to you will surprise you.

Not only do you develop the existing senses by such practice and use, *but you help in the unfoldment of the latent powers and senses that are striving for unfoldment*. By using and exercising the faculties that we have, we help to unfold those for the coming of which we have been dreaming.

MANTRAM (AFFIRMATION)

I am a Soul, possessed of channels of communication with the outer world. I will use these channels, and thereby acquire the information and knowledge necessary for my mental development. I will exercise and develop my organs of sense, knowing that in so doing I shall cause to unfold the higher senses, of which they are but forerunners and symbols. I will be "*wide-awake*" and open to the inflow of knowledge and information. The Universe is my Home—I will explore it.

THE SEVENTH LESSON

THE UNFOLDMENT OF CONSCIOUSNESS.

We have thought it well to make a slight change in the arrangement of these lessons—that is, in the order in which they should appear. We had contemplated making this Seventh Lesson a series of Mental Drills, intended to develop certain of the mental faculties, but we have decided to postpone the same until a later lesson, believing that by so doing a more logical sequence or order of arrangement will be preserved. In this lesson we will tell you of the unfoldment of consciousness in Man, and in the next lesson, and probably in the one following it, we shall present to you a clear statement regarding the states of mind, below and over consciousness—a most wonderful region, we assure you, and one that has been greatly misunderstood and misinterpreted.

This will lead up to the subject of the cultivation of the various faculties—both conscious and outside of consciousness, and the series will be concluded by three lessons going right to the heart of this part of the subject, and giving certain rules and instruction calculated to develop Man's wonderful "thought-machine" that will be of the greatest interest and importance to all of our students. When the lessons are concluded you will see that the present arrangement is most logical and proper.

In this lesson we take up the subject of "The Unfoldment of Consciousness"—a most interesting subject. Many of us have been in the habit of identifying "consciousness" with mind, but as we proceed with this series of lessons, we will see that that which is called "consciousness" is but a small portion of the mind of the individual, and even that small part is constantly changing its states, and unfolding new states undreamed of.

"Consciousness" is a word we use very often in considering the science of the Mind. Let us see what it means. Webster defines it as one's "knowledge of sensations and mental operations, or of what passes in one's own mind." Halleck defines it as "that undefinable characteristic of mental states which causes one to be aware of them." But, as Halleck states, "Consciousness is incapable of definition. To define anything, we are obliged to describe it in terms of something else. And there is nothing else in the world like consciousness, hence we can define it only in terms of itself, and that is very much like trying to lift one's self by one's own boot straps. Consciousness is one of the greatest mysteries that confronts us."

Before we can understand what Consciousness really is, we must know just what "Mind" really is—and that knowledge is lacking, notwithstanding the many ingenious theories evolved in order to explain the mystery. The metaphysicians do not throw much light on the subject, and as for materialistic science, listen to what Huxley says: "How it comes about that anything so remarkable as a state of consciousness comes about by the result of irritating nervous tissue, is just as unaccountable as the appearance of the genie when Aladdin rubbed his lamp."

To many persons the words "consciousness" and "mental process," or "thought" are regarded as synonymous. And, in fact, psychologists so held until quite recently. But now it is generally accepted as a fact that mental processes are not limited to the field of consciousness, and it is now generally taught that the field of sub-consciousness (that is, "under" conscious) mentation, is of a much greater extent than that of conscious mentation.

Not only is it true that the mind can hold in consciousness but one fact at any one instant, and that, consequently, only a very small fraction of our knowledge can be in consciousness at any one moment, but it is also true that the consciousness plays but a very small part in the totality of mental processes, or mentation. The mind is not conscious of the greater portion of its own activities—Maudsley says that only ten per cent comes into the field of consciousness. Taine has stated it in these words: "Of the world which makes up our being, we only perceive the highest points—the lighted up peaks of a continent whose lower levels remain in the shade."

But it is not our intention to speak of this great subconscious region of the mind at this point, for we shall have much to do with it later on. It is mentioned here in order to show that the enlargement or development of consciousness is not so much a matter of "growth" as it is an "unfoldment"—not a new creation or enlargement from outside, but rather an unfoldment outward from within.

From the very beginning of Life—among the Particles of Inorganic Substance, may be found traces of something like Sensation, and response thereto. Writers have not cared to give to this phenomenon the name of "sensation," or "sensibility," as the terms savored too much of "senses," and "sense-organs." But Modern Science has not hesitated to bestow the names so long withheld. The most advanced scientific writers do not hesitate to state that in reaction, chemical response, etc., may be seen indications of rudimentary sensation. Haeckel says: "I cannot imagine the simplest chemical and physical process without attributing the movement of the material particles to unconscious sensation. The idea of Chemical Affinity consists in the fact that the various chemical elements perceive the qualitative differences in other elements and experience 'pleasure' or 'revulsion' at contacts with them, and execute their specific movements on this ground." He also speaks of the sensitiveness of "plasm," or the substance of "living bodies," as being "only a superior degree of the general irritability of substance."

Chemical reaction, between atoms, is spoken of by chemists as a "sensitive" reaction. Sensitiveness is found even in the Particles of Inorganic Substance, and may be regarded as the first glimmerings of thought. Science recognizes this when it speaks of the unconscious sensation of the Particles as *athesis* or "feeling," and the unconscious Will that responds thereto, as *tropesis*, or "inclination." Haeckel says of this that "Sensation perceives the different qualities of the stimuli, and feeling the quantity," and also, "We may ascribe the feeling of pleasure and pain (in the contact with qualitatively differing atoms) to all atoms, and so explain the elective affinity in chemistry (attraction of loving atoms, inclination; repulsion of hating atoms, disinclination)."

It is impossible to form a clear or intelligent idea of the phenomenon of chemical affinity, etc., unless we attribute to the Atoms something akin to Sensation. It is likewise impossible to understand the actions of the Molecules, unless we think of them as possessing something akin to Sensation. The Law of Attraction is based upon Mental States in Substance. The response of Inorganic Substance to Electricity and Magnetism is also another evidence of Sensation and the response thereto.

In the movements and operations of crystal-life we obtain evidences of still a little higher form of Sensation and response thereto. The action of crystallization is very near akin to that of some low forms of plasmic action. In fact, the "missing link" between plant life and the crystals is claimed to have been found in some recent discoveries of Science, the connection being found in certain crystals in the interior of plants composed of carbon combinations, and resembling the inorganic crystals in many ways.

Crystals grow along certain lines and forms up to a certain size. Then they begin to form "baby-crystals" on their surfaces, which then take on the growth—the processes being almost analogous to cell-life. Processes akin to fermentation have been detected among chemicals. In many ways it may be seen that the beginning of Mental Life must be looked for among the Minerals and Particles—the latter, be it remembered, composing not only inorganic, but also Organic Substance.

As we advance in the scale of life, we are met with constantly increasing unfoldment of mentation, the simple giving place to the complex manifestations. Passing by the simple vital processes of the monera, or single-celled "things," we notice the higher forms of cell life, with growing sensibility or sensation. Then we come to the cell-groups, in which the individual cells manifest sensation of a kind, coupled with a community-sensation. Food is distinguished, selected and captured, and movements exercised in pursuit of the same. The living thing is beginning to manifest more complex mental states. Then the stage of the lower plants is reached, and we notice the varied phenomena of that region, evidencing an increased sensitiveness, although there are practically no signs of special organs of sense. Then we pass on to the higher plant life, in which begin to manifest certain "sensitive-cells," or groups of such cells, which are rudimentary sense organs. Then the forms of animal life, and considered with rising degrees of sensations and growing sense apparatus, or sense organs, gradually unfolding into something like nervous systems.

Among the lower animal forms there are varying degrees of mentation with accompanying nerve centers and sense-organs, but little or no signs of consciousness, gradually ascending until we have dawning consciousness in the reptile kingdom, etc., and fuller consciousness and a degree of intelligent thought in the still higher forms, gradually increasing until we reach the plane of the highest mammals, such as the horse, dog, elephant, ape, etc., which animals have complex nervous systems, brains and well developed consciousness. We need not further consider the forms of mentation in the forms of life below the Conscious stage, for that would carry us far from our subject.

Among the higher forms of animal life, after a "dawn period" or semi-consciousness, we come to forms of life among the lower animals possessing a well-developed degree of mental action and Consciousness, the latter being called by psychologists "Simple Consciousness," but which term we consider too indefinite, and which we will term "Physical Consciousness," which will give a fair idea of the thing itself. We use the word "Physical" in the double sense of "External," and "Relating to the material structure of a living being," both of which definitions are found in the dictionaries.

And that is just what Physical Consciousness really is—an "awareness" in the mind, or a "consciousness" of the "external" world as evidenced by the senses; and of the "body" of the animal or person. The animal or person thinking on the plane of Physical Consciousness (all the higher animals do, and many men seem unable to rise much higher) identifies itself with the physical body, and is conscious only of thoughts of that body and the outside world.

It "knows," but not being conscious of mental operations, or of the existence of its mind, it does not "know that it knows." This form of consciousness, while infinitely above the mentation of the nonconscious plane of "sansation," is like a different world of thought from the consciousness of the highly developed intellectual man of our age and race.

It is difficult for a man to form an idea of the Physical Consciousness of the lower animals and savages, particularly as he finds it difficult to understand his own consciousness except by the act of being conscious. But observation and reason have given us a fair degree of understanding of what this Physical Consciousness of the animal is like—or at least in what respect it differs from our own consciousness. Let us take a favorite illustration. A horse standing out in the cold sleet and rain undoubtedly *feels* the discomfort, and possibly pain, for we know by observation that animals feel both. But he is not able to analyze his mental states and wonder when his master will come out to him—think how cruel it is to keep him out of the warm stable—wonder whether he will be taken out in the cold again tomorrow—feel envious of other horses who are indoors—wonder why he is compelled to be out cold nights, etc., etc.

In short, he does not think as would a reasoning man under such circumstances. He is aware of the discomfort, just as would be the man—and he would run home if he could just as would the man. But he is not able to pity himself, nor to think about his personality as would the man, nor does he wonder whether such a life is worth living, after all. He "knows," but is not able to think of himself as knowing—he does not "know that he knows," as we do. He experiences the physical pain and discomfort, but is spared the mental discomfort and concern arising from the physical, which man so often experiences.

The animal cannot shift its consciousness from the sensations of the outer world to the inner states of being. It is not able to "know itself." The difference may be clumsily illustrated by the example of a man feeling, seeing or hearing something that gives him a pleasurable sensation, or the reverse. He is conscious of the feeling or sensation, and that it is pleasurable or otherwise. That is Physical Consciousness, and the animal may share it with him.

But it stops right there with the animal. But the man may begin to wonder *why* the sensation is pleasurable and to associate it with other things and persons; or speculate *why* he dislikes it, what will follow, and so on—that is Mental Consciousness, because he recognizes an inward self, and is turning his attention *inward*. He may see another man and experience a feeling or sensation of attraction or aversion—like or dislike. This is Physical Consciousness, and an animal also may experience the sensation. But the man goes further than the animal, and wonders just what there is about the man he likes or detests, and may compare himself to the man and wonder whether the latter feels as he does, and so on—this is Mental Consciousness.

In animals the mental gaze is freely directed outward, and never returns upon itself. In man the mental gaze may be directed inward, or may return inward after its outward journey. The animal "knows"—the man not only "knows," but he "knows that he knows," and is able to investigate that "knowing" and speculate about it. We call this higher consciousness Mental Consciousness. The operation of Physical Consciousness we call Instinct—the operation of Mental Consciousness we call Reason.

The Man who has Mental Consciousness not only "feels" or "senses" things, but he has words or mental concepts of these feelings and sensations and may think of himself as experiencing them, separating himself, the sensation or feeling, and the thing felt or sensed. The man is able to think: "I feel; I hear; I see; I smell; I taste; I desire; I do," etc., etc. The very words indicate Mental Consciousness recognizing mental states and giving them names, and also recognizing something called "I" that experiences the sensations. This latter fact has caused psychologists to speak of this stage as "Self-consciousness," but we reserve this idea of the "I" consciousness for a higher stage.

The animal experiences something that gives it the impressions or feeling that we call "pain," "hurt," "pleasant," "sweet," "bitter," etc., all being forms of sensation, but it is unable to think of them in words. The pain seems to be a part of itself, although possibly associated with some person or thing that caused it. The study of the unfoldment of consciousness in a young baby will give one a far better idea of the grades and distinctions than can be obtained from reading mere words.

Mental Consciousness is a growth. As Halleck says, "Many persons never have more than a misty idea of such a mental attitude. They always take themselves for granted, and never turn the gaze inward." It has been doubted whether the savages have developed Self-consciousness, and even many men of our own race seem to be but little above the animals in intellect and consciousness. They do not seem able to "know themselves" even slightly. To them the "I" seems to be a purely physical thing—a body having desires and feeling but little more. They are able to feel an act, but scarcely more. They are not able to set aside any physical "not—I," being utterly unable to think of themselves as anything else but a Body. The "I" and the Body are one with them, and they seem incapable of distinguishing between them.

Then comes another stage in which mental-consciousness proper sets in. The man begins to realize that he has "a mind." He is able to "know himself" as a mental being, and to turn the gaze inward a little. This period of development may be noticed in young children. For a time, they speak of themselves as a third person, until finally they begin to say "I." Then a little later comes the ability to know their own mental states as such—they know that they have a mind, and are able to distinguish between it and the body. It is related that some children experience a feeling of terror when they pass into this stage. They exhibit signs of bashfulness and what is commonly termed "self-consciousness" in that sense. Some tell us in after years that when they became aware of themselves as an entity they were overcome with alarm, as if by a sense of loneliness and apartness from the Universe. Young people often feel this way for several years. There seems to be a distinct feeling that the Universe is antagonistic to and set apart from them.

And, although this feeling of separateness and apartness grows less acute as the man grows older, yet it is always present to a greater or less degree until a still higher stage—the Ego-consciousness is reached, when it disappears as we shall see. And this mental-conscious stage is a hard one for many. They are entangled in a mass of mental states which the man thinks is "himself," and the struggle between the real "I" and its confining sheaths is painful. And it becomes still more painful as the end is neared, for as man advances in mental-consciousness and knowledge he feels more keenly and suffers accordingly. Man eats the fruit of the Tree of Knowledge and begins to suffer, and is driven out of the Garden of Eden of the child and primitive races, who live like the birds of the air and concern themselves not about mental states and problems. But there is deliverance ahead in the shape of a higher consciousness, although but few realize it and still fewer have gained it. Perhaps this lesson may point out the way for you.

With the birth of mental-consciousness comes the knowledge that there is a mind in others. Man is able to speculate and reason about the mental states of other men, because he recognizes these states within himself. As man advances in the Mental Consciousness, he begins to develop a constantly increasing degree and grade of Intellect, and accordingly he attaches the greatest importance to that part of his nature. Some men worship Intellect as a God, ignoring its limitations which other thinkers have pointed out. Such people are apt to reason that because the human intellect (in its present state of development) reports that such a thing *must* be, or *cannot* possibly be, that the matter is forever settled.

They ignore the fact that it is possible that Man's Intellect, in its present state of unfoldment, may be able to take cognizance of only a very small part of the Universal Fact, and that there may be regions upon regions of Reality and Fact of which he cannot even dream, so far are they removed from his experience. The unfoldment of a new sense would open out a new world and might bring to light facts that would completely revolutionize our entire world of conceptions by reason of the new information it would give us.

But, nevertheless, from this Mental Consciousness has come the wonderful work of Intellect, as shown in the achievements of Man up to this time, and while we must recognize its limitations, we gladly join in singing its praises. Reason is the tool with which Man is digging into the mine of Facts, bringing to light new treasures every day. This stage of Mental Consciousness is bringing to Man knowledge of himself—knowledge of the Universe—that is well worth the price he pays for it. For Man *does* pay a price for entrance into this stage—and he pays an increasing price as he advances in its territory, for the higher he advances the more keenly he feels and suffers, as well as enjoys.

Capacity for pain is the price Man pays for Attainment, up to a certain stage. His pain passes from the Physical to the Mental consciousness, and he becomes aware of problems that he never dreamt existed, and the lack of an intelligent answer produces mental suffering. And the mental suffering that comes to him from unsatisfied longings, disappointment, the pain of others whom he loves, etc., is far worse than any physical suffering.

The animal lives its animal life and is contented, for it knows no better. If it has enough to eat—a place to sleep—a mate—it is happy. And some men are likewise. But others find themselves involved in a world of mental discomfort. New wants arise, and the lack of satisfaction brings pain. Civilization becomes more and more complex, and brings its new pains as well as new pleasures. Man attaches himself to "things," and each day creates for himself artificial wants, which he must labor to meet. His Intellect may not lead him upward, but instead may merely enable him to invent new and subtle means and ways of gratifying his senses to a degree impossible to the animals. Some men make a religion of the gratification of their sensuality—their appetites—and become beasts magnified by the power of Intellect. Others become vain, conceited and puffed up with a sense of the importance of their Personality (the false "I").

Others become morbidly introspective, and spend their time analyzing and dissecting their moods, motives, feelings, etc. Others exhaust their capacity for pleasure and happiness, but looking outside for it instead of within, and become *blasé*, bored, *ennuied* and an affliction to themselves We mention these things not in a spirit of Pessimism but merely to show that even this great Mental Consciousness has a reverse and ugly side as well as the bright face that has been ascribed to it.

As man reaches the higher stages of this Mental Consciousness, and the next higher stage begins to dawn upon him, he is apt to feel more keenly than ever the insufficiency of Life as it appears to him. He is unable to understand Himself—his origin, destiny, purpose and nature—and he chafes against the bars of the cage of Intellect in which he is confined. He asks himself the question, "Whence come I—Whither go I—What is the object of my Existence?" He becomes dissatisfied with the answers the world has to give him to these questions, and he cries aloud in despair—and but the answer of his own voice comes back to him from the impassable walls with which he is surrounded. He does not realize that his answer must come from Within—but so it is.

Psychology stops when it reaches the limits of Mental Consciousness, or as it calls it "Self-Consciousness," and denies that there is anything beyond—any unexplored regions of the Mind. It laughs at the reports that come from those who have penetrated farther within the recesses of their being, and dismisses the reports as mere "dreams," "fantasies," "illusions," "ecstatic imaginings," "abnormal states," etc., etc. But, nevertheless, there are schools of thought that teach of these higher states, and there are men of all ages and races that have entered them and have reported concerning them. And we feel justified in asking you to take them into consideration.

There are two planes of Consciousness, of which we feel it proper to speak, for we have obtained more or less information regarding them. There are still higher planes, but they belong to higher phases of life than are dealt with here.

The first of these planes or states of Consciousness, above the "Self-Consciousness" of the psychologists (which we have called "Mental Consciousness") may be called "Ego-consciousness," for it brings an "awareness" of the Reality of the Ego. This "awareness" is far above the Self-consciousness of the man who is able to distinguish "I" from "You," and to give it a name. And far above the consciousness that enables a man, as he rises in the scale, to distinguish the "I" from faculty after faculty of the mind, which he is able to recognize as "not—I," until he finds left a mental something that he cannot set aside, which he calls "I"—although this stage alone is very much higher than that of the average of the race, and is a high degree of Attainment itself.

It is akin to this last stage, and yet still fuller and more complete. In the dawning of Ego Consciousness, the "I" recognizes itself still more clearly and, more than this, is fully imbued with a sense and "awareness" of its own *Reality*, unknown to it before. This awareness is not a mere matter of reasoning—it is a "consciousness," just as is Physical Consciousness and Mental Consciousness something different from an "intellectual conviction." It is a Knowing, not a Thinking or Believing. The "I" *knows* that it is Real—that it has its roots in the Supreme Reality underlying all the Universe, and partakes of its Essence. It does not know what this Reality is, but it knows that it is Real, and something different from anything in the world of name, form, number, time, space, cause and effect—something Transcendental and surpassing all human experience. And knowing this, it knows that it cannot be destroyed or hurt; cannot die, but is immortal; and that there is Something which is the very essence of Good behind of, underneath and even *in* itself. And in this certainty and consciousness is their Peace, Understanding and Power. When it fully bursts upon one, Doubt, Fear, Unrest and Dissatisfaction drop from him like worn-out garments and he finds himself clothed in the Faith that Knows; Fearlessness; Restfulness; Satisfaction. Then he is able to say understandingly and with meaning "I AM."

This Ego Consciousness is coming to many as a dawning knowledge—the light is just rising from behind the hills. To others it has come gradually and slowly, but fully, and they now live in the full light of the consciousness. Others it has burst upon like a flash, or vision—like a light falling from the clear sky, almost blinding them at first, but leaving them changed men and women, possessed of that something that cannot be understood by or described to those who have not experienced it. This last stage is called "Illumination" in one of its forms.

The man of the Ego Consciousness may not understand the Riddle of the Universe or be able to give an answer to the great Questions of Life—but he has ceased to worry about them—they now disturb him not. He may use his intellect upon them as before, but never with the feeling that in their intellectual solution rests his happiness or peace of mind. He knows that he stands on solid rock, and though the storms of the world of matter and force may beat upon him, he will not be hurt. This and other things he knows. He cannot prove these things to others, for they are not demonstrable by argument—he himself did not get them in that way.

And so, he says but little about it—but lives his life as if he knew them not, so far as outward appearances go. But inwardly he is a changed man—his life is different from that of his brothers, for while their souls are wrapped in slumber or are tossing in troubled dreams, his Soul has awakened and is gazing upon the world with bright and fearless eyes. There are, of course, different stages or degrees of this Consciousness, just as there are in the lower planes of consciousness. Some have it to a slight degree, while others have it fully. Perhaps this lesson will tell some of its readers just what is the thing that has "happened" to them and which they hesitate to speak of to their closest friend or life companion. To others it may open the way to a fuller realization. We sincerely trust so, for one does not begin to Live until he knows the "I" as Reality.

There is a stage still higher than this last mentioned but it has come to but very few of the race. Reports of it come from all times, races, countries. It has been called "Cosmic Consciousness," and is described as an awareness of the Oneness of Life—that is, a consciousness that the Universe is filled with One Life—an actual perception and "awareness" that the Universe is full of Life, Motion and Mind, and that there is no such thing as Blind Force, or Dead Matter, but that All is alive, vibrating and intelligent. That is, of course, that the *Real Universe*, which is the Essence or background of the Universe of Matter, Energy and Mind, is as they describe.

In fact, the description of those who have had glimpses of this state would indicate that they see the Universe as All Mind—that All is Mind at the last. This form of consciousness has been experienced by men here and there—only a few—in moments of "Illumination," the period lasting but a very short space of time, then fading away, leaving but a memory. In the moment of the "Illumination" there came to those experiencing it a sense of "intouch-ness" with Universal Knowledge and Life, impossible to describe, accompanied by a Joy beyond understanding.

Regarding this last, "Cosmic Consciousness," we would state that it means more than an intellectual conviction, belief or realization of the facts as stated, for an actual *vision* and *consciousness* of these things came in the moment of Illumination. Some others report that they have a deep abiding sense of the reality of the facts described by the report of the Illumined, but have not experienced the "vision" or ecstasy referred to. These last people seem to have with them always the same mental state as that possessed by those who had the "vision" and passed out of it, carrying with them the remembrance and feeling, but not the actual consciousness attained at the moment.

They agree upon the essential particulars of the reports. Dr. Maurice Bucke, now passed out of this plane of life, wrote a book entitled "Cosmic Consciousness," in which he describes a number of these cases, including his own, Walt Whitman's and others, and in which he holds that this stage of consciousness is before the race and will gradually come to it in the future. He holds that the manifestation of it which has come to some few of the race, as above stated, is but the first beams of the sun which are flashing upon us and which are but prophecies of the appearance of the great body of light itself.

We shall not here consider at length the reports of certain great religious personages of the past, who have left records that in moments of great spiritual exaltation they became conscious of "being in the presence of the Absolute," or perhaps within the radius of "the light of Its countenance." We have great respect for these reports, and have every reason for believing many of them authentic, notwithstanding the conflicting reports that have been handed down to us by those experiencing them. These reports are conflicting because of the fact that the minds of those who had these glimpses of consciousness were not prepared or trained to fully understand the nature of the phenomena. They found themselves in the spiritual presence of Something of awful grandeur and spiritual rank, and were completely dazed and bewildered at the sight.

They did not understand the nature of the Absolute, and when they had sufficiently recovered, they reported that they had been in the "presence of God"—the word "God" meaning their particular conception of Deity—that is, the one appearing as Deity in their own particular religious creed or school. They saw nothing to cause them to identify this Something with their particular conception of Deity, except that they thought that "it *must* be God," and knowing no other God except their own particular conception, they naturally identifying the Something with "God" as they conceived Him to be. And their reports naturally were along these lines.

Thus, the reports of all religions are filled with accounts of the so-called miraculous occurrences. The Catholic saint reports that he "saw of light of God's countenance," and the non-Catholic reports likewise regarding God as he knows him. The Mohammedan reports that he caught a glimpse of the face of Allah, and the Buddhist tells us that he saw Buddha under the tree. The Brahman has seen the face of Brahma, and the various Hindu sects have men who give similar reports regarding their own particular deities. The Persians have given similar reports, and even the ancient Egyptians have left records of similar occurrences. These conflicting reports have led to the belief, on the part of those who did not understand the nature of the phenomena, that these things were "all imagination" and fancy, if indeed not rank falsehood and imposture. But the Yogis know better than this.

They know that underneath all these varying reports there is a common ground of truth, which will be apparent to anyone investigating the matter. They know that all of these reports (except a few based upon fraudulent imitation of the real phenomenon) are based upon truth and are but the bewildered reports of the various observers. They know that these people were temporarily lifted above the ordinary plane of consciousness and were made aware of the existence of a Being or Beings higher than mortal.

It does not follow that they saw "God" or the Absolute, for there are many Beings of high spiritual growth and development that would appear to the ordinary mortal as a very God. The Catholic doctrine of Angels and Arch-angels is corroborated by those among the Yogis who have been "behind the Veil," and they give us reports of the "Devas" and other advanced Beings. So, the Yogi accepts these reports of the various mystics, saints and inspired ones, and accounts for them all by laws perfectly natural to the students of the Yogi Philosophy, but which appear as supernatural to those who have not studied along these lines.

But we cannot speak further of this phase of the subject in this lesson, for a full discussion of it would lead us far away from the phase of the general subject before us. But we wish to be understood as saying that there are certain centers in the mental being of Man from which may come light regarding the existence of the Absolute and higher order of Beings. In fact, from these centers come to man that part of his mental "feelings" that he calls "the religious instinct or intuition." Man does not arrive at that underlying consciousness of "Something Beyond" by means of his Intellect—it is the glimmer of light coming from the higher centers of the Self.

He notices these gleams of light, but not understanding them, he proceeds to erect elaborate theological and creedal structures to account for them, the work of the Intellect, however, always lacking that "feeling" that the intuition itself possesses. True religion, no matter under what name it may masquerade, comes from the "heart" and is not comforted or satisfied with these Intellectual explanations, and hence comes that unrest and craving for satisfaction which comes to Man when the light begins to break through.

But we must postpone a further discussion of this part of the subject for the present. We shall consider it again in a future lesson in connection with other matters. As we have said, our next two lessons will take upon the inquiry regarding the regions outside of the consciousness of the ordinary man. You will find it a most fascinating and instructive inquiry and one that will open up new fields of thought for many of you.

MANTRAM (AFFIRMATION)

I Am a Being far greater and grander than I have as yet conceived. I am unfolding gradually but surely into higher planes of consciousness. I am moving Forward and Upward constantly. My goal is the Realization of the True Self, and I welcome each stage of Unfoldment that leads me toward my aim. I am a manifestation of REALITY. I *AM*.

THE EIGHTH LESSON

THE HIGHLANDS AND LOWLANDS OF MIND.

The Self of each of us has a vehicle of expression which we call the Mind, but which vehicle is much larger and far more complex than we are apt to realize. As a writer has said "Our Self is greater than we know; it has peaks above, and lowlands below the plateau of our conscious experience." That which we know as the "conscious mind" is not the Soul. The Soul is not a part of that which we know in consciousness, but, on the contrary, that which we know in consciousness is but a small part of the Soul—the conscious vehicle of a greater Self, or "I."

The Yogis have always taught that the mind has many planes of manifestation and action—and that many of its planes operated above and below the plane of consciousness. Western science is beginning to realize this fact, and its theories regarding same may be found in any of the later works on psychology. But this is a matter of recent development in Western science. Until very recently the text books held that Consciousness and Mind were synonymous, and that the Mind was conscious of all of its activities, changes and modifications.

Liebnitz was one of the first Western philosophers to advance the idea that there were planes of mental activity outside of the plane of consciousness, and since his time the leading thinkers have slowly but surely moved forward to his position.

At the present time it is generally conceded that at least ninety per cent of our mental operations take place in the out-of-conscious realm. Prof. Elmer Gates, the well-known scientist, has said: "At least ninety per cent of our mental life is sub-conscious. If you will analyze your mental operations you will find that conscious thinking is never a continuous line of consciousness, but a series of conscious data with great intervals of subconscious. We sit and try to solve a problem, and fail. We walk around, try again, and fail. Suddenly an idea dawns that leads to the solution of the problem. The subconscious processes were at work. We do not volitionally create our own thinking. It takes place in us. We are more or less passive recipients. We cannot change the nature of a thought, or of a truth, but we can, as it were, *guide the ship by a moving of the helm*. Our mentation is largely the result of the great Cosmic Whole upon us."

Sir William Hamilton says that the sphere of our consciousness is only a small circle in the center of a far wider sphere of action and thought, of which we are conscious through its effects.

Taine says: "Outside of a little luminous circle, lies a large ring of twilight, and beyond this an indefinite night; but the events of this twilight and this night are as real as those within the luminous circle."

Sir Oliver Lodge, the eminent English scientist, speaking of the planes of the mind, says: "Imagine an iceberg glorying in its crisp solidity, and sparkling pinnacles, resenting attention paid to its submerged self, or supporting region, or to the saline liquid out of which it arose, and into which in due course it will someday return. Or, reversing the metaphor, we might liken our present state to that of the hulls of ships submerged in a dim ocean among strange monsters, propelled in a blind manner through space; proud perhaps of accumulating many barnacles as decoration; only recognizing our destination by bumping against the dock-wall; and with no cognizance of the deck and cabins above us, or the spars and sails—no thought of the sextant, and the compass, and the captain—no perception of the lookout on the mast—of the distant horizon. With no vision of objects far ahead—dangers to be avoided—destinations to be reached—other ships to be spoken to by means other than by bodily contact—a region of sunshine and cloud, of space, or perception, and of intelligence utterly inaccessible to parts below the waterline."

We ask our students to read carefully the above expression of Sir Oliver Lodge, for it gives one of the clearest and most accurate figures of the actual state of affairs concerning the mental planes that we have seen in Western writings.

And other Western writers have noted and spoken of these out-of-conscious realms. Lewes has said: "It is very certain that in every conscious volition—every act that is so characterized—the larger part of it is quite unconscious. It is equally certain that in every perception there are unconscious processes of reproduction and inference. There is a middle distance of sub-consciousness, and a background of unconsciousness."

Taine has told us that: "Mental events imperceptible to consciousness are far more numerous than the others, and of the world that makes up our being we only perceive the highest points—the lighted-up peaks of a continent whose lower levels remain in the shade. Beneath ordinary sensations are their components, that is to say, the elementary sensations, which must be combined into groups to reach our consciousness."

Maudsley says: "Examine closely and without bias the ordinary mental operations of daily life, and you will find that consciousness has not one-tenth part of the function therein which it is commonly assumed to have. In every conscious state there are at work conscious, sub-conscious, and infra-conscious energies, the last as indispensable as the first."

Oliver Wendall Holmes said: "There are thoughts that never emerge into consciousness, which yet make their influence felt among the perceptible mental currents, just as the unseen planets sway the movements of those that are watched and mapped by the astronomer."

Many other writers have given us examples and instances of the operation of the out-of-consciousness planes of thought. One has written that when the solution of a problem he had long vainly dealt with, flashed across his mind, he trembled as if in the presence of another being who had communicated a secret to him. All of us have tried to remember a name or similar thing without success, and have then dismissed the matter from our minds, only to have the missing name or thought suddenly presented to our conscious mind a few minutes, or hours, afterwards. Something in our mind was at work hunting up the missing word, and when it found it it presented it to us.

A writer has mentioned what he called "unconscious rumination," which happened to him when he read books presenting new points of view essentially opposed to his previous opinions. After days, weeks, or months, he found that to his great astonishment the old opinions were entirely rearranged, and new ones lodged there. Many examples of this unconscious mental digestion and assimilation are mentioned in the books on the subject written during the past few years.

It is related of Sir W. R. Hamilton that he discovered quarternions one day while walking with his wife in the observatory at Dublin. He relates that he suddenly felt "the galvanic circle of thought" close, and the sparks that fell from it was the fundamental mathematical relations of his problem, which is now an important law in mathematics.

Dr. Thompson has written: "At times I have had a feeling of the uselessness of all voluntary effort, and also that the matter was working itself clear in my mind. It has many times seemed to me that I was really a passive instrument in the hands of a person not myself. In view of having to wait for the results of these unconscious processes, I have proved the habit of getting together material in advance, and then leaving the mass to digest itself till I am ready to write about it. I delayed for a month the writing of my book 'System of Psychology,' but continued reading the authorities. I would not try to think about the book. I would watch with interest the people passing the windows. One evening when reading the paper, the substance of the missing part of the book flashed upon my mind, and I began to write. This is only a sample of many such experiences."

Berthelot, the founder of Synthetic Chemistry has said that the experiments leading to his wonderful discoveries have never been the result of carefully followed trains of thought—of pure reasoning processes—but have come of themselves, so to speak, from the clear sky.

Mozart has written: "I cannot really say that I can account for my compositions. My ideas flow, and I cannot say whence or how they come. I do not hear in my imagination the parts successively, but I hear them, as it were, all at once. The rest is merely an attempt to reproduce what I have heard."

Dr. Thompson, above mentioned, has also said: "In writing this work I have been unable to arrange my knowledge of a subject for days and weeks, until I experienced a clearing up of my mind, when I took my pen and unhesitatingly wrote the result. I have best accomplished this by leading the (conscious) mind as far away as possible from the subject upon which I was writing."

Prof. Barrett says: "The mysteriousness of our being is not confined to subtle physiological processes which we have in common with all animal life. There are higher and more capacious powers wrapped up in our human personality than are expressed even by what we know of consciousness, will, or reason. There are supernormal and transcendental powers of which, at present, we only catch occasional glimpses; and behind and beyond the supernormal there are fathomless abysses, the Divine ground of the soul; the ultimate reality of which our consciousness is but the reflection or faint perception. Into such lofty themes I do not propose to enter, they must be forever beyond the scope of human inquiry; nor is it possible within the limits of this paper to give any adequate conception of those mysterious regions of our complex personality, which are open to, and beginning to be disclosed by, scientific investigation."

Rev. Dr. Andrew Murray has written: "Deeper down than where the soul with its consciousness can enter there is spirit matter linking man with God; and deeper down than the mind and feelings or will—in the unseen depths of the hidden life—there dwells the Spirit of God." This testimony is remarkable, coming from that source, for it corroborates and reiterates the Yogi teachings of the Indwelling Spirit Schofield has written: "Our conscious mind as compared with the unconscious mind, has been likened to the visible spectrum of the sun's rays, as compared to the invisible part which stretches indefinitely on either side. We know now that the chief part of heat comes from the ultra-red rays that show no light; and the main part of the chemical changes in the vegetable world are the results of the ultra-violet rays at the other end of the spectrum, which are equally invisible to the eye, and are recognized only by their potent effects. Indeed as these invisible rays extend indefinitely on both sides of the visible spectrum, so we may say that the mind includes not only the visible or conscious part, and what we have termed the sub-conscious, that which lies below the red line, but the supraconscious mind that lies at the other end—all those regions of higher soul and spirit life, of which we are only at times vaguely conscious, but which always exist, and link us on to eternal verities, on the one side, as surely as the sub-conscious mind links us to the body on the other."

We know that our students will appreciate the above testimony of Dr. Schofield, for it is directly in the line of our teachings in the Yogi Philosophy regarding the Planes of the Mind (see "Fourteen Lessons").

We feel justified in quoting further from Dr. Schofield, for he voices in the strongest manner that which the Yogi Philosophy teaches as fundamental truths regarding the mind. Dr. Schofield is an English writer on Psychology, and so far as we know has no tendency toward occultism, his views having been arrived at by careful scientific study and investigation along the lines of Western psychology, which renders his testimony all the more valuable, showing as it does, how the human mind will instinctively find its way to the Truth, even if it has to blaze a new trail through the woods, departing from the beaten tracks of other minds around it, which lack the courage or enterprise to strike out for themselves.

Dr. Schofield writes: "The mind, indeed, reaches all the way, and while on the one hand it is inspired by the Almighty, on the other it energizes the body, all whose purposive life it originates. We may call the supra-conscious mind the sphere of the spirit life, the sub-conscious the sphere of the body life, and the conscious mind the middle region where both meet."

Continuing, Dr. Schofield says: "The Spirit of God is said to dwell in believers, and yet, as we have seen, His presence is not the subject of direct consciousness. We would include, therefore, in the supra-conscious, all such spiritual ideas, together with conscience—the voice of God, as Max Muller calls it—which is surely a half-conscious faculty. Moreover, the supra-conscious, like the sub-conscious, is, as we have said, best apprehended when the conscious mind is not active. Visions, meditations, prayers, and even dreams have been undoubtedly occasions of spiritual revelations, and many instances may be adduced as illustrations of the workings of the Spirit apart from the action of reason or mind. The truth apparently is that the mind as a whole is an unconscious state, by that its middle registers, excluding the highest spiritual and lowest physical manifestations, are fitfully illuminated in varying degree by consciousness; and that it is to this illuminated part of the dial that the word "mind," which rightly appertains to the whole, has been limited."

Oliver Wendell Holmes has said: "The automatic flow of thought is often singularly favored by the fact of listening to a weak continuous discourse, with just enough ideas in it to keep the (conscious) mind busy. The induced current of thought is often rapid and brilliant in inverse ratio to the force of the inducing current."

Wundt says: "The unconscious logical processes are carried on with a certainty and regularity which would be impossible where there exists the possibility of error. Our mind is so happily designed that it prepares for us the most important foundations of cognition, whilst we have not the slightest apprehension of the *modus operandi*. This unconscious soul, like a benevolent stranger, works and makes provisions for our benefit, pouring only the mature fruits into our laps."

A writer in an English magazine interestingly writes: "Intimations reach our consciousness from unconsciousness, that the mind is ready to work, is fresh, is full of ideas." "The grounds of our judgment are often knowledge so remote from consciousness that we cannot bring them to view." "That the human mind includes an unconscious part; that unconscious events occurring in that part are proximate causes of consciousness; that the greater part of human intuitional action is an effect of an unconscious cause; the truth of these propositions is so deducible from ordinary mental events, and is so near the surface that the failure of deduction to forestall induction in the discerning of it may well excite wonder."

"Our behavior is influenced by unconscious assumptions respecting our own social and intellectual rank, and that of the one we are addressing. In company we unconsciously assume a bearing quite different from that of the home circle. After being raised to a higher rank the whole behavior subtly and unconsciously changes in accordance with it." And Schofield adds to the last sentence: "This is also the case in a minor degree with different styles and qualities of dress and different environments. Quite unconsciously we change our behavior, carriage, and style, to suit the circumstance."

Jensen writes: "When we reflect on anything with the whole force of the mind, we may fall into a state of entire unconsciousness, in which we not only forget the outer world, but also know nothing at all of ourselves and the thoughts passing within us after a time. We then suddenly awake as from a dream, and usually at the same moment the result of our meditations appears as distinctly in consciousness without our knowing how we reached it."

Bascom says: "It is inexplicable how premises which lie below consciousness can sustain conclusions in consciousness; how the mind can wittingly take up a mental movement at an advanced stage, having missed its primary steps."

Hamilton and other writers have compared the mind's action to that of a row of billiard balls, of which one is struck and the impetus transmitted throughout the entire row, the result being that only the last ball actually moves, the others remaining in their places. The last ball represents the conscious thought—the other stages in the unconscious mentation. Lewes, speaking of this illustration, says: "Something like this, Hamilton says, seems often to occur in a train of thought, one idea immediately suggesting another into consciousness—this suggestion passing through one or more ideas which do not themselves rise into consciousness. This point, that we are not conscious of the formation of groups, but only of a formed group, may throw light on the existence of unconscious judgments, unconscious reasonings, and unconscious registrations of experience."

Many writers have related the process by which the unconscious mentation emerges gradually into the field of consciousness, and the discomfort attending the process. A few examples may prove interesting and instructive.

Maudsley says: "It is surprising how uncomfortable a person may be made by the obscure idea of something which he ought to have said or done, and which he cannot for the life of him remember. There is an effort of the lost idea to get into consciousness, which is relieved directly the idea bursts into consciousness."

Oliver Wendell Holmes said: "There are thoughts that never emerge into consciousness, and which yet make their influence felt among the perceptive mental currents, just as the unseen planets sway the movements of the known ones." The same writer also remarks: "I was told of a business man in Boston who had given up thinking of an important question as too much for him. But he continued so uneasy in his brain that he feared he was threatened with palsy. After some hours the natural solution of the question came to him, worked out, as he believed, in that troubled interval."

Dr. Schofield mentions several instances of this phase of the workings of the unconscious planes of the mind. We mention a couple that seem interesting and to the point:

"Last year," says Dr. Schofield, "I was driving to Phillmore Gardens to give some letters to a friend. On the way, a vague uneasiness sprang up, and a voice seemed to say, 'I doubt if you have those letters.' Conscious reason rebuked it, and said, 'Of course you have; you took them out of the drawer specially.' The vague feeling was not satisfied, but could not reply. On arrival I found the letters were in none of my pockets. On returning I found them on the hall table, where they had been placed a moment putting on my gloves."

"The other day I had to go to see a patient in Folkestone, in Shakespeare Terrace. I got there very late, and did not stay but drove down to the Pavilion for the night, it being dark and rainy. Next morning at eleven I walked up to find the house, knowing the general direction, though never having walked there before. I went up the main road, and, after passing a certain turning, began to feel a vague uneasiness coming into consciousness, that I had passed the terrace. On asking the way, I found it was so; and the turning was where the uneasiness began. The night before was pitch dark, and very wet, and anything seen from a close carriage was quite unconsciously impressed on my mind."

Prof. Kirchener says: "Our consciousness can only grasp one quite clear idea at once. All other ideas are for the time somewhat obscure. They are really existing, but only potentially for consciousness, *i.e.,* they hover, as it were, on our horizon, or beneath the threshold of consciousness. The fact that former ideas suddenly return to consciousness is simply explained by the fact that they have continued psychic existence: and attention is sometimes voluntarily or involuntarily turned away from the present, and the appearance of former ideas is thus made possible."

Oliver Wendell Holmes says: "Our different ideas are stepping-stones; how we get from one to another we do not know; something carries us. We (our conscious selves) do not take the step. The creating and informing spirit, which is *within* us and not *of* us, is recognized everywhere in real life. It comes to us as a voice that will be heard; it tells us what we must believe; it frames our sentences and we wonder at this visitor who chooses our brain as his dwelling place."

Galton says: "I have desired to show how whole states of mental operation that have lapsed out of ordinary consciousness, admit of being dragged into light."

Montgomery says: "We are constantly aware that feelings emerge unsolicited by any previous mental state, directly from the dark womb of unconsciousness. Indeed, all our most vivid feelings are thus mystically derived. Suddenly a new irrelevant, unwilled, unlooked-for presence intrudes itself into consciousness. Some inscrutable power causes it to rise and enter the mental presence as a sensorial constituent. If this vivid dependence on unconscious forces has to be conjectured with regard to the most vivid mental occurrences, how much more must such a sustaining foundation be postulated for those faint revivals of previous sensations that so largely assist in making up our complex mental presence!"

Sir Benjamin Brodie says: "It has often happened to me to have accumulated a store of facts, but to have been able to proceed no further. Then after an interval of time, I have found the obscurity and confusion to have cleared away: the facts to have settled in their right places, though I have not been sensible of having made any effort for that purpose."

Wundt says: "The traditional opinion that consciousness is the entire field of the internal life cannot be accepted. In consciousness, psychic acts are very distinct from one another, and observation itself necessarily conducts to unity in psychology. But the agent of this unity is outside of consciousness, which knows only the result of the work done in the unknown laboratory beneath it. Suddenly a new thought springs into being. Ultimate analysis of psychic processes shows that the unconscious is the theater of the most important mental phenomena. The conscious is always conditional upon the unconscious."

Creighton says: "Our conscious life is the sum of these entrances and exits. Behind the scenes, as we infer, there lies a vast reserve which we call 'the unconscious,' finding a name for it by the simple device of prefixing the negative article. The basis of all that lies behind the scene is the mere negative of consciousness."

Maudsley says: "The process of reasoning adds nothing to knowledge (in the reasoner). It only displays what was there before, and brings to conscious possession what before was unconscious." And again: "Mind can do its work without knowing it. Consciousness is the light that lightens the process, not the agent that accomplishes it."

Walstein says: "It is through the sub-conscious self that Shakespeare must have perceived, without effort, great truths which are hidden from the conscious mind of the student; that Phidias painted marble and bronze; that Raphael painted Madonnas, and Beethoven composed symphonies."

Ribot says: "The mind receives from experience certain data, and elaborates them unconsciously by laws peculiar to itself, and the result merges into consciousness."

Newman says: "When the unaccustomed causes surprise, we do not perceive the thing and then feel the surprise; but surprise comes first, and then we search out the cause; so, the theory must have acted on the unconscious mind to create the feeling, before being perceived in consciousness."

A writer in an English magazine says: "Of what transcendent importance is the fact that the unconscious part of the mind bears to the conscious part such a relation as the magic lantern bears to the luminous disc which it projects; that the greater part of the intentional action, the whole practical life of the vast majority of men, is an effect of events as remote from consciousness as the motion of the planets."

Dr. Schofield says: "It is quite true that the range of the unconscious mind must necessarily remain indefinite; none can say how high or low it may reach.... As to how far the unconscious powers of life that, as has been said, can make eggs and feathers out of Indian corn, and milk and beef and mutton out of grass, are to be considered within or beyond the lowest limits of unconscious mind, we do not therefore here press. It is enough to establish the fact of its existence; to point out its more important features; and to show that in all respects it is as worthy of being called mind as that which works in consciousness. We therefore return to our first definition of Mind, as 'the sum of psychic action in us, whether conscious or unconscious.'"

Hartmann calls our attention to a very important fact when he says: "The unconscious does not fall ill, the unconscious does not grow weary, but all conscious mental activity becomes fatigued."

Kant says: "To have ideas and yet not be conscious of them—therein seems to lie a contradiction. However, we may still be immediately aware of holding an idea, though we are not directly conscious of it."

Maudsley says: "It may seem paradoxical to assert not merely that ideas may exist in the mind without any consciousness of them, but that an idea, or a train of associated ideas, may be quickened into action and actuate movements without itself being attended to. When an idea disappears from consciousness it does not necessarily disappear entirely; it may remain latent below the horizon of consciousness. Moreover, it may produce an effect upon movement, or upon other ideas, when thus active below the horizon of consciousness."

Liebnitz says: "It does not follow that because we do not perceive thought that it does not exist. It is a great source of error to believe that there is no perception in the mind but that of which it is conscious."

Oliver Wendell Holmes says: "The more we examine the mechanism of thought the more we shall see that anterior unconscious action of the mind that enters largely into all of its processes. People who talk most do not always think most. I question whether persons who think most—that is who have most conscious thought pass through their mind—necessarily do most mental work. Every new idea planted in a real thinker's mind grows when he is least conscious of it."

Maudsley says: "It would go hard with mankind indeed, if they must act wittingly before they acted at all. Men, without knowing why, follow a course for which good reasons exist. Nay, more. The practical instincts of mankind often work beneficially in actual contradiction to their professed doctrines."

The same writer says: "The best thoughts of an author are the unwilled thoughts which surprise himself; and the poet, under the influence of creative activity, is, so far as consciousness is concerned, being dictated to."

A writer in an English magazine says: "When waiting on a pier for a steamer, I went on to the first, which was the wrong one. I came back and waited, losing my boat, which was at another part of the pier, on account of the unconscious assumption I had made, that this was the only place to wait for the steamer. I saw a man enter a room, and leave by another door. Shortly after, I saw another man exactly like him do the same. It was the same man; but I said it must be his twin brother, in the unconscious assumption that there was no exit for the first man but by the way he came (that by returning)."

Maudsley says: "The firmest resolve or purpose sometimes vanishes issueless when it comes to the brink of an act, while the true will, which determines perhaps a different act, springs up suddenly out of the depths of the unconscious nature, surprising and overcoming the conscious."

Schofield says: "Our unconscious influence is the projection of our unconscious mind and personality unconsciously over others. This acts unconsciously on their unconscious centers, producing effects in character and conduct, recognized in consciousness. For instance, the entrance of a good man into a room where foul language is used, will unconsciously modify and purify the tone of the whole room. Our minds cast shadows of which we are as unconscious as those cast by our bodies, but which affect for good or evil all who unconsciously pass within their range. This is a matter of daily experience, and is common to all, though more noticeable with strong personalities."

Now we have given much time and space to the expressions of opinion of various Western writers regarding this subject of there being a plane or planes of the mind outside of the field of consciousness. We have given space to this valuable testimony, not alone because of its intrinsic value and merit, but because we wished to impress upon the minds of our students that these out-of-conscious planes of mind are now being recognized by the best authorities in the Western world, although it has been only a few years back when the idea was laughed at as ridiculous, and as a mere "dream of the Oriental teachers." Each writer quoted has brought out some interesting and valuable point of the subject, and the student will find that his own experiences corroborate the points cited by the several writers. In this way we think the matter will be made plainer, and will become fixed in the mind of those who are studying this course of lessons.

But we must caution our students from hastily adopting the several theories of Western writers, advanced during the past few years, regarding these out-of-conscious states. The trouble has been that the Western writers dazzled by the view of the subconscious planes of mentation that suddenly burst upon the Western thought, hastily adopted certain theories, which they felt would account for all the phenomena known as "psychic," and which they thought would fully account for all the problems of the subject. These writers while doing a most valuable work, which has helped thousands to form new ideas regarding the nature and workings of the mind, nevertheless did not sufficiently explore the nature of the problem before them. A little study of the Oriental philosophies might have saved them and their readers much confusion.

For instance, the majority of these writers hastily assumed that because there *was* an out-of-conscious plane of mentation, therefore all the workings of the mind might be grouped under the head of "conscious" and "sub-conscious," and that all the out-of-conscious phenomena might be grouped under the head of "subconscious mind," "subjective mind," etc., ignoring the fact that this class of mental phenomena embraced not only the highest but the lowest forms of mentation In their newly found "mind" (which they called "subjective" or "sub-conscious"), they placed the lowest traits and animal passions; insane impulses; delusions; bigotry; animal-like intelligence, etc., etc., as well as the inspiration of the poet and musician, and the high spiritual longings and feelings that one recognizes as having come from the higher regions of the soul.

This mistake was a natural one, and at first reading the Western world was taken by storm, and accepted the new ideas and theories as Truth. But when reflection came, and analysis was applied there arose a feeling of disappointment and dissatisfaction, and people began to feel that there was something lacking. They intuitively recognized that their higher inspirations and intuitions came from a different part of the mind than the lower emotions, passions, and other sub-conscious feelings, and instincts.

A glance at the Oriental philosophies will give one the key to the problem at once. The Oriental teachers have always held that the conscious mentation was but a small fraction of the entire volume of thought, but they have always taught that just as there was a field of mentation *below* consciousness, so was there a field of mentation *above* consciousness as much higher than Intellect as the other was lower than it. The mere mention of this fact will prove a revelation to those who have not heard it before, and who have become entangled with the several "dual-mind" theories of the recent Western writers. The more one has read on this subject the more he will appreciate the superiority of the Oriental theory over that of the Western writers. It is like the chemical which at once clears the clouded liquid in the test-tube.

In our next lesson we shall go into this subject of the above-conscious planes, and the below-conscious planes, bringing out the distinction clearly, and adding to what we have said on the subject in previous books.

And all this is leading us toward the point where we may give you instruction regarding the training and cultivation—the retraining and guidance of these out-of-conscious faculties. By retraining the lower planes of mentation to their proper work, and by stimulating the higher ones, man may "make himself over." mentally, and may acquire powers of which he but dreams now. This is why we are leading you up to the understanding of this subject, step by step. We advise you to acquaint yourself with each phase of the matter, that you may be able to apply the teachings and instructions to follow in later lessons of the course.

MANTRAM (AFFIRMATION)

I recognize that my Self is greater than it seems—that above and below consciousness are planes of mind—that just as there are lower planes of mind which belong to my past experience in ages past and over which I must now assert my Mastery—so are there planes of mind into which I am unfolding gradually, which will bring me wisdom, power, and joy. I Am Myself, in the midst of this mental world—I am the Master of my Mind—I assert my control of its lower phases, and I demand of its higher all that it has in store for me.

THE NINTH LESSON

THE MENTAL PLANES.

In our last lesson we told you something about the operation of the mind outside of the field of consciousness. In this lesson we will attempt to classify these out-of-consciousness planes, by directing your attention to the several mental planes above and below the plane of consciousness. As we stated in the last lesson, over 90 per cent of our mental operations are conducted outside of the field of consciousness, so that the consideration of the planes is seen to be an important subject.

Man is a Centre of Consciousness in the great One Life of the Universe. His soul has climbed a great many steps before it reached its present position and stage of unfoldment. And it will pass through many more steps until it is entirely free and delivered from the necessity of its swaddling clothes.

In his mental being man contains traces of all that has gone before—all the experiences of himself and the great race movement of which he is a part. And, likewise, his mind contains faculties and mental planes which have not as yet unfolded into consciousness, and of the existence of which he is but imperfectly aware. All of these mental possessions, however, are useful and valuable to him—even the lowest. The lowest may be used to advantage, under proper mastery, and are only dangerous to the man who allows them to master him instead of serving him as they should, considering his present stage of development.

In this consideration of the several mental planes we shall not confine ourselves to the technical occult terms given to these several planes, but will place them in general groups and describe the features and characteristics of each, rather than branch off into long explanations of the growth and reason of the several planes, which would take us far away from the practical consideration of the subject.

Beginning at the lowest point of the scale we see that man has a body. The body is composed of minute cells of protoplasm. These cells are built up of countless molecules, atoms and particles of matter—precisely the same matter that composes the rocks, trees, air, etc., around him. The Yogi philosophy tells us that even the atoms of matter have life and an elementary manifestation of mind, which causes them to group together according to the law of attraction, forming different elements, combinations, etc. This law of attraction is a mental operation, and is the first evidence of mental choice, action and response. Below this is Prana or Force, which, strictly speaking, is also a manifestation of mind, although for convenience we designate it as a separate manifestation of the Absolute.

And therefore, we find that this law of attraction between the atoms and particles of matter is a mental action, and that it belongs to man's mental kingdom, because he has a body and this mental action is continually going on in his body. So therefore, this is the lowest mental plane to be considered in the make-up of the man. This plane is, of course, far sunken beneath the plane of consciousness, and is scarcely identified with the personality of the man at all, but rather belongs to the life of the whole, manifest in the rock as well as in the man.

But after these atoms have been grouped by the law of attraction and have formed molecules of matter, they are taken possession of by a higher mental activity and built up into cells by the mental action of the plant. The life impulse of the plant begins by drawing to it certain particles of inorganic matter—chemical elements—and then building them into a single cell. Oh, mystery of the cell! The intellect of man is unable to duplicate this wonderful process. The Mind Principle on the Vegetative Plane, however, knows exactly how to go to work to select and draw to itself just the elements needed to build up the single cell. Then taking up its abode in that cell—using it as a basis of operations, it proceeds to duplicate its previous performance, and so cell after cell is added, by the simple reproductive process of division and subdivision—the primitive and elemental sex process—until the mighty plant is built up. From the humblest vegetable organism up to the greatest oak the process is the same.

And it does not stop there. The body of man is also built up in just this way, and he has this vegetative mind also within him, below the plane of consciousness, of course. To many this thought of a vegetative mind may be somewhat startling. But let us remember that every part of our body has been built up from the vegetable cell. The unborn child starts with the coalition of two cells. These cells begin to build up the new body for the occupancy of the child—that is, the mind principle in the cells directs the work, of course—drawing upon the body of the mother for nourishment and supplies. The nourishment in the mother's blood, which supplies the material for the building up of the child's body, is obtained by the mother eating and assimilating the vegetable cells of plants, directly or indirectly. If she eats fruit, nuts, vegetables, etc., she obtains the nourishment of the plant life directly—if she eats meat, she obtains it indirectly, for the animal from which the meat was taken built up the meat from vegetables. There is no two ways about this—all nourishment of the animal and human kingdom is obtained from the vegetable kingdom, directly or indirectly.

And the cell action in the child is identical with the cell action in the plant. Cells constantly reproducing themselves and building themselves up into bodily organs, parts, etc., under the direction and guidance of the mind principle. The child grows in this way until the hour of birth. It is born, and then the process is but slightly changed. The child begins to take nourishment either from the mother's milk or from the milk of the cow, or other forms of food. And as it grows larger it partakes of many different varieties of food. But always it obtains building material from the cell life of the plants.

And this great building up process is intelligent, purposeful, to a wonderful degree. Man with his boasted intellect cannot explain the real "thingness" of the process. A leading scientist who placed the egg of a small lizard under microscopical examination and then watched it slowly develop has said that it seemed as if some hand was tracing the outlines of the tiny vertebrae, and then building up around it. Think for a moment of the development of the germ within the egg of the humming-bird, or the ant, or the gnat, or the eagle. Every second a change may be noticed. The germ cell draws to itself nourishment from the other part of the egg, and then it grows and reproduces another cell. Then both cells divide—then subdivide until there are millions and millions and millions of cells. And all the while the building up process continues, and the bird or insect assumes shape and form, until at last the work is accomplished and the young bird emerges from the egg.

And the work thus commenced continues until the death of the animal. For there is a constant using-up and breaking-down of cell and tissue, which the organism must replace. And so the vegetative mind of the plant, or insect, or animal, or man, is constantly at work building up new cells from the food, throwing out worn-out and used-up material from the system. Not only this, but it attends to the circulation of the blood in order that the materials for the building up may be carried to all parts of the system. It attends to the digestion and assimilation of the food—the wonderful work of the organs of the body.

It attends to the healing of wounds, the fight against disease, the care of the physical body. And all this out of the plane of consciousness—in the infant man the animal world, the vegetable kingdom—ever at work, untiring, intelligent, wonderful. And this plane of mind is in man as well as in the plant, and it does its work without aid from the conscious part of man, although man may interfere with it by adverse conscious thought, which seems to paralyze its efforts. Mental Healing is merely the restoring of normal conditions, so that this part of the body may do its work without the hindrance of adverse conscious thought.

On this plane of the mind is found all of the vital functions and operations. The work is done out-of-consciousness, and the consciousness is aware of this part of the mind only when it makes demands upon the conscious for food, etc. On this plane also resides the elementary instinct that tends toward reproduction and sexual activity. The demand of this part of the mind is always "increase and multiply," and according to the stage of growth of the individual is the mandate carried out, as we shall see presently. The elementary impulses and desires that we find rising into the field of consciousness come from this plane of the mind. Hunger, thirst and the reproductive desires are its messages to the higher parts of the mind.

And these messages are natural and free from the abuses and prostitution often observed attached to them by the intellect of man in connection with his unrestrained animal impulses. Gluttony and unnatural lust arise not from the primitive demand of this plane of the mind—for the lower animals even are free from them to a great extent—but it is reserved for man to so prostitute these primitive natural tendencies, in order to gratify unnatural and artificial appetites, which serve to frustrate nature rather than to aid her.

As Life advanced in the scale and animal forms appeared on the scene new planes of mind were unfolded, in accordance to the necessity of the living forms. The animal was compelled to hunt for his food—to prey upon other forms, and to avoid being preyed upon by others. He was compelled to struggle for the unfoldment of latent powers of his mind that would give him means to play his part in the scheme of life. He was compelled to do certain things in order to live and reproduce his kind. And he demanded not in vain. For there came to him slowly an unfolding knowledge of the things necessary for the requirements of his life. We call this Instinct.

But, pray remember, by Instinct we do not mean the still higher something that is really rudimentary Intellect that we notice in the higher animals. We are speaking now of the unreasoning instinct observed in the lower animals, and to a certain degree in man. This Instinctive plane of mentality causes the bird to build its nest before its eggs are laid, which instructs the animal mother how to care for its young when born, and after birth; which teaches the bee to construct its cell and to store up its honey. These and countless other things in animal life, and in the higher form of plant life, are manifestations of Instinct—that great plane of the mind. In fact, the greater part of the life of the animal is instinctive although the higher forms of animals have developed something like rudimentary Intellect or Reason, which enables them to meet new conditions where Intellect alone fails them.

And man has this plane of mind within him, below consciousness. In fact, the lower forms of human life manifest but little Intellect, and live almost altogether according to their Instinctive impulses and desires.

Every man has this Instinctive mental region within him and from it are constantly arising impulses and desires to perplex and annoy him, as well as to serve him occasionally. The whole secret consists in whether the man has Mastery of his lower self or not.

From this plane of the mind arise the hereditary impulses coming down from generations of ancestors, reaching back to the cavemen, and still further back into the animal kingdom. A queer storehouse is this. Animal instincts—passions, appetites, desires, feelings, sensations, emotions, etc., are there. Hate, envy, jealousy, revenge, the lust of the animal seeking the gratification of his sexual impulses, etc., etc., are there, and are constantly intruding upon our attention until we have asserted our mastery. And often the failure to assert this mastery comes from an ignorance of the nature of the desire, etc.

We have been taught that these thoughts were "bad" without being told *why*, and we have feared them and thought them the promptings of an impure nature, or a depraved mind, etc. This is all wrong. These things are not "bad" of themselves—they came to us honestly—they are our heritage from the past. They belong to the animal part of our nature, and were necessary to the animal in his stage of development. We have the whole menagerie within us, but that does not mean that we should turn the beasts loose upon ourselves or others. It was necessary for the animal to be fierce, full of fight, passionate, regardless of the rights of others, etc., but we have outgrown that stage of development, and it is ignoble for us to return to it, or to allow it to master us.

This lesson is not intended as a discourse upon Ethics or morals. We do not intend going into a discussion of the details of "Right and Wrong," for we have touched upon that phase of the subject in other works. But we feel justified in calling your attention to the fact that the human mind intuitively recognizes the "Rightness" of the living up to that which comes to us from the highest parts of the mind—the highest product of our unfoldment. And it likewise intuitively recognizes the "Wrongness" of the falling back into that which belongs to the lower stages of our mentality—to the animal part of us, that is our heritage from the past and that which has gone before.

While we may be puzzled about many details of morals and ethics and may not be able to "explain" why we consider certain things right or wrong, we still intuitively feel that the highest "Right" of which we are capable is the acting out of that which is coming to us from the highest pole of our mental being, and that the lowest "Wrong" consists in doing that which carries us back to the life of the lower animals, in so far as mentality is concerned. Not because there is anything absolutely "Wrong" in the mental processes and consequent of the animals in themselves—they are all right and perfectly natural in the animals—but we intuitively recognize that for us to fall back to the animal stage is a "going backward" in the scale of evolution. We intuitively shrink at an exhibition of brutality and animality on the part of a man or woman. We may not know just why, but a little reflection will show us that it is a sinking in the evolutionary scale, against which the spiritual part of us revolts and protests.

But this must not be construed to mean that the advanced soul looks upon the animal world with disgust or horror. On the contrary, there is nowhere to be found a higher respect for animal life and being than among the Yogi and other advanced souls. They delight in watching the animals filling their places in life—playing out their parts in the divine scheme of life. Their animal passions and desires are actions viewed sympathetically and lovingly by the advanced soul, and nothing "Wrong" or disgusting is seen there. And even the coarseness and brutality of the savage races are so regarded by these advanced souls. They see everything as natural according to the grade and degree of development of these people.

It is only when these advanced souls view the degeneracies of "civilized" life that they feel sorrow and pain. For here they see instances of devolution instead of evolution—degeneration instead of regeneration and advancement. And not only do they know this to be the fact, but the degenerate specimens of mankind themselves feel and know it. Compare the expression of the animal or savage going through their natural life actions and performances. See how free and natural are their expressions, how utterly apart are evidences of wrong doing.

They have not as yet found out the fatal secret of Good and Evil—they have not as yet eaten the forbidden fruit. But, on the contrary, look into the faces of the degenerates and fallen souls of our civilized life. See the furtive glance and the self-consciousness of "Wrong" evident in every face. And this consciousness of "Wrong" bears heavily upon these people—it is heavier than the punishments heaped upon them That nameless something called "conscience" may be smothered for a while, but sooner or later it comes to light and demands the pound of flesh from its victim.

And yet you will say that it seems hard to think that the same thing can be Right in one person and Wrong in another. This seems like a hard saying and a dangerous doctrine, but it is the Truth. And man instinctively recognizes it. He does not expect the same sense of moral responsibility in a young child, or in a savage, that he does in a mature, developed, civilized man. He may restrain the child and the savage, for self-protection and the welfare of all, but he realizes the distinction, or at least should do so. And not only is this true, but as man advances in the scale, he casts off many ideas of "Wrong" that he once held, having outgrown the old ideas and having grown into new conceptions. And the tendency is always upward and onward. The tendency is constantly from Force and Restraint toward Love and Freedom. The ideal condition would be one in which there were no laws and no necessity for them—a condition in which men had ceased to do wrong because they had outgrown the desire rather than from fear or restraint or force. And while this condition as yet seems afar off, there is constantly going on an unfoldment of higher planes and faculties of the mind, which when once fully manifest in the race will work a complete revolution in ethics and laws and government—and for the better, of course. In the meantime, Mankind moves along, doing the best it can, making a steady though slow progress.

There is another plane of the mind which is often called the "Instinct," but which is but a part of the plane of the Intellect, although its operations are largely below the field of consciousness. We allude to what may be called the "Habit Mind," in order to distinguish it from the Instinctive Plane. The difference is this: The Instinctive plane of mind is made up of the ordinary operations of the mind below the plane of the Intellect, and yet above the plane of the Vegetative mind—and also of the acquired experiences of the race, which have been transmitted by heredity, etc. But the "Habit Mind" contains only that which has been placed there by the person himself and which he has acquired by experience, habit, and observation, repeated so often until the mind knows it so well that it is carried below the field of consciousness and becomes "second nature," and akin to Instinct.

The text books upon psychology are filled with illustrations and examples of the habit phase or plane of the mental operations, and we do not think it necessary to repeat instances of the same kind here. Everyone is familiar with the fact that tasks which at first are learned only by considerable work and time soon become fixed in some part of the mind until their repetition calls for little or no exercise of conscious mental operation. In fact, some writers have claimed that no one really "learns" how to perform a task until he can perform it almost automatically.

The pupil who in the early stages of piano playing finds it most difficult to control and manage his fingers, after a time is able to forget all about his fingering and devote his entire attention to the pages of his music, and after this he is able to apparently let his fingers play the entire piece of music by themselves without a thought on his part. The best performers have told us that in the moments of their highest efforts they are aware that the out-of-conscious portion of their mind is doing the work for them, and they are practically standing aside and witnessing the work being done. So true is this that in some cases it is related that if the performer's conscious mind attempts to take up the work the quality is impaired and the musician and the audience notice the difference.

The same thing is true in the case of the woman learning to operate the sewing machine. It is quite difficult at first, but gradually it grows to "run itself." Those who have mastered the typewriter have had the same experience. At first each letter had to be picked out with care and effort. After a gradual improvement the operator is enabled to devote her entire attention to the "copy" and let the fingers pick out the keys for themselves.

Many operators learn rapid typewriting by so training the habit mind that it picks out the letter-keys by reason of their position, the letters being covered over in order to force the mind to adapt itself to the new requirements. A similar state of affairs exists wherever men or women have to use tools of any kind. The tool soon is recognized by the mind and used as if it were a part of the body, and no more conscious thought is devoted to the manipulation than we devote to the operation of walking, which, by the way, is learned by the child only by the expenditure of time and labor. It is astonishing how many things we do "automatically" in this way. Writers have called our attention to the fact that the average man cannot consciously inform you how he puts on his coat in the morning—which arm goes in first, how the coat is held, etc. But the habit mind knows—knows very well. Let the student stand up and put on his coat in the regular way, following the leadings of the habit mind.

Then, after removing it, let him attempt to put it on by inserting the other arm first, for instance. He will be surprised to find out how awkward it will be for him, and how completely he has been depending upon the habit mind. And tomorrow morning let him find out which shoe the habit mind has been putting on him first and then try to reverse the order and notice how flurried and disturbed the habit mind will become, and how frantically it will signal to the conscious mind: "Something wrong up there!" Or try to button on your collar, reversing the order in which the tabs are placed over the button—right before left, or left before right, as the case may be, and notice the involuntary protest. Or, try to reverse the customary habit in walking and attempt to swing your right arm with the movement of your right leg, and so on, and you will find it will require the exercise of great will power. Or, try to "change hands" and use your knife and fork. But we must stop giving examples and illustrations. Their number is countless.

Not only does the habit mind attend to physical actions, etc., but it also takes a hand in our mental operations. We soon acquire the habit of ceasing to consciously consider certain things, and the habit mind takes the matter for granted, and thereafter we will think automatically on those particular questions, unless we are shaken out of the habit by a rude jolt from the mind of someone else, or from the presentation of some conflicting idea occasioned by our own experience or reasoning processes. And the habit mind hates to be disturbed and compelled to revise its ideas. It fights against it, and rebels, and the result is that many of us are slaves to old outgrown ideas that we realize are false and untrue, but which we find that we "cannot exactly get rid of." In our future lessons we will give methods to get rid of these old outgrown ideas.

There are other planes of mind which have to do with the phenomena known as "psychic," by which is meant the phases of psychic phenomena known as clairvoyance, psychometry, telepathy, etc., but we shall not consider them in this lesson, for they belong to another part of the general subject. We have spoken of them in a general way in our "Fourteen Lessons in Yogi Philosophy, etc."

And now we come to the plane of mind known to us as Intellect or the Reasoning Faculties. Webster defines the word Intellect as follows: The part or faculty of the human soul by which it knows, as distinguished from the power to feel and to will; the thinking faculty; the understanding. The same authority defines the word Reason as follows: "The faculty or capacity of the human mind by which it is distinguished from the intelligence of the inferior animals." We shall not attempt to go into a consideration of the conscious Intellect, for to do so we would be compelled to take up the space of the remaining lessons of the course, and besides, the student may find extended information on this subject in any of the text books on psychology. Instead, we will consider other faculties and planes of mind which the said text books pass by rapidly, or perhaps deny. And one of these planes is that of Unconscious Reasoning, or Intellect. To many this term will seem paradoxical, but students of the unconscious will understand just what is meant.

Reasoning is not necessarily conscious in its operations, in fact, a greater part of the reasoning processes are performed below or above the conscious field. In our last lesson we have given a number of examples proving this fact, but a few more remarks may not be out of place, nor without interest to the student.

In our last lesson you will see many instances stated in which the sub-conscious field of the Intellect worked out problems, and then after a time handed to the conscious reason the solution of the matter. This has occurred to many of us, if not indeed to all of us. Who has not endeavored to solve a problem or question of some sort and after "giving it up" has had it suddenly answered and flashed into consciousness when least expected. The experience is common to the race. While the majority of us have noticed these things, we have regarded them as exceptional and out of the general rule. Not so, however, with students of the mental planes. The latter have recognized these planes of reason, and have availed themselves of their knowledge by setting these unconscious faculties to work for them. In our next lesson we will give directions to our students regarding this accomplishment, which may prove of the greatest importance to those who will take the trouble to practice the directions given. It is a plan that is known to the majority of men who have "done things" in the world, the majority of them, however, having discovered the plan for themselves as the result of a need or demand upon the inner powers of mind.

The plane of mind immediately above that of Intellect is that known as Intuition. Intuition is defined by Webster as follows: "Direct apprehension or cognition; immediate knowledge, as in perception or consciousness, involving no reasoning process; quick or ready insight or apprehension." It is difficult to explain just what is meant by Intuition, except to those who have experienced it—and these people do not need the explanation. Intuition is just as real a mental faculty as is Intellect—or, to be more exact, is just as much a collection of mental faculties. Intuition is above the field of consciousness, and its messages are passed downward, though its processes are hidden. The race is gradually unfolding into the plane of Intuition, and the race will some day pass into full consciousness on that plane.

In the meantime, it gets but flashes and glimpses from the hidden region. Many of the best things we have come from that region. Art, music, the love of the beautiful and good poetry, the higher form of love, spiritual insight to a certain degree, intuitive perception of truth, etc., etc., come from this region. These things are not reasoned out by the intellect, but seem to spring full born from some unknown region of the mind.

In this wonderful region dwells Genius. Many, if not all of the great writers, poets, musicians, artists and other examples of genius have felt that their power came to them from some higher source. Many have thought that it emanated from some being kindly to them, who would inspire them with power and wisdom. Some transcendent power seemed to have been called into operation, and the worker would feel that his product or creation was not his handiwork, but that of some outside intelligence. The Greeks recognized this something in man, and called it man's "Daemon." Plutarch in his discourse on the daemon that guided Socrates speaks of the vision of Timarchus, who, in the case of Trophonius, saw spirits which were partly attached to human bodies, and partly over and above them, shining luminously over their heads. He was informed by the oracle that the part of the spirit which was immersed in the body was called the "soul," but that the outer and unimmersed portion was called the "daemon." The oracle also informed him that every man had his daemon, whom he is bound to obey; those who implicitly follow that guidance are the prophetic souls, the favorites of the gods. Goethe also spoke of the daemon as a power higher than the will, and which inspired certain natures with miraculous energy.

We may smile at these conceptions, but they are really very close to the truth. The higher regions of the mind, while belonging to the individual, and a part of himself, are so far above his ordinary consciousness that to all intents and purposes messages from them are as orders from another and higher soul. But still the voice is that of the "I," speaking through its sheaths as best it is able.

This power belongs to every one of us, although it manifests only in the degree that we are able to respond to it. It grows by faith and confidence, and closes itself up, and withdraws into its recesses when we doubt it and would question its veracity and reality. What we call "originality" comes from this region. The Intuitive faculties pass on to the conscious mind some perception of truth higher than the Intellect has been able to work out for itself, and lo! it is called the work of genius.

The advanced occultist knows that in the higher regions of the mind are locked up intuitive perceptions of all truth, and that he who can gain access to these regions will know everything intuitively, and as a matter of clear sight, without reasoning or explanation. The race has not as yet reached the heights of Intuition—it is just beginning to climb the foothills. But it is moving in the right direction. It will be well for us if we will open ourselves to the higher inner guidance, and be willing to be "led by the Spirit."

This is a far different thing from being led by outside intelligence, which may, or may not, be qualified to lead. But the Spirit within each of us has our interests at heart and is desirous of our best good, and is not only ready but willing to take us by the hand and lead us on. The Higher Self is doing the best it can for our development and welfare, but is hampered by the confining sheaths. And alas, many of us glory in these sheaths and consider them the highest part of ourselves. Do not be afraid to let the light of the Spirit pierce through these confining sheaths and dissolve them. The Intuition, however, is not the Spirit, but is one of its channels of communication to us. There are other and still higher planes of mind, but the Intuition is the one next in the line of unfoldment, and we should open ourselves to its influence and welcome its unfoldment.

Above the plane of Intuition is that of the Cosmic Knowing, upon which we will find the consciousness of the Oneness of All. We have spoken of this plane in our lesson on the Unfoldment of Consciousness. When one is able to "conscious" on this plane—this exalted plane of mind—he is able to see fully, plainly and completely that there is One Great Life underlying all the countless forms and shapes of manifestation. He is able to see that separateness is only "the working fiction of the Universe." He is able to see that each Ego is but a Centre of Consciousness in the great Ocean of Life—all in pursuance of the Divine Plan, and that he is moving forward toward higher and higher planes of manifestation, power and individuality, in order to take a greater and grander part in the Universal work and plans.

The Cosmic Knowing in its fulness has come to but few of the race, but many have had glimpses, more or less clear, of its transcendent wonder, and others are on the borderland of this plane. The race is unfolding gradually, slowly but surely, and those who have had this wonderful experience are preparing others for a like experience. The seed is being sown, and the harvest will come later. This and other phases of the higher forms of consciousness are before the race. The individuals who read this lesson are perhaps nearer to it than they think; their interest in the lessons is an indication of that hunger of the soul which is a prophecy of the satisfaction of the cry for spiritual bread. The Law of Life heeds these cries for aid and nourishment and responds accordingly, but along the lines of the highest wisdom and according to the *real requirements* of the individual.

Let us close this lesson with a quotation from "Light on the Path," which bears directly upon the concluding thought. Read it carefully and let it sink down deep into your inner consciousness, and you will feel the thrill of joy that comes to him who is nearing the goal.

"Look for the flower to bloom in the silence that follows the storm; not till then.

"It shall grow, it will shoot up, it will make branches and leaves, and form buds while the storm lasts. But not until the entire personality of the man is dissolved and melted—not until it is held by the divine fragment which has created it, as a mere subject for grave experiment and experience—not until the whole nature has yielded and become subject unto its higher self, can the bloom open. Then will come a calm such as comes in a tropical country after the heavy rain, when nature works so swiftly that one may see her action. Such a calm will come to the harassed spirit. And in the deep silence the mysterious event will occur which will prove that the way has been found. Call it by whatever name you will. It is a voice that speaks where there is none to speak, it is a messenger that comes—a messenger without form or substance—or it is the flower of the soul that has opened. It cannot be described by any metaphor. But it can be felt after, looked for, and desired, even among the raging of the storm. The silence may last a moment of time, or it may last a thousand years. But it will end. Yet you will carry its strength with you. Again and again the battle must be fought and won. It is only for an interval that nature can be still."

The concluding three lessons of this series will be devoted to a practical course of instruction in the development of the hidden planes of the mind, or rather, in the development of the power of the individual to master the same and make use of them in his life. He will be taught to master the lower principles, not only in the surmounting of them, but in the transmitting of the elemental forces toward his higher ends. Power may be obtained from this part of the mind, under the direction of the Will. And the student will be told how to set the unconscious Intellect to work for him. And he will be told how to develop and train the Will. We have now passed the line between the theoretical and the practical phases of the subject, and from now on it will be a case of train, develop, cultivate and apply. Knowing what lies back of it all, the student is now prepared to receive the instructions which he might have misused before. Peace be with thee all.

MANTRAM (AFFIRMATION)

I AM THE MASTER OF MY SOUL.

THE TENTH LESSON

SUB-CONSCIOUSING.

In the Ninth Lesson we called your attention to the fact that Reasoning was not necessarily conscious in its operations, and that, in fact, a large part of the rational processes of the mind are performed below or above the field of consciousness. And in the Eighth Lesson we gave you a number of examples illustrating this fact. We also gave you a number of cases in which the sub-conscious field of the Intellect worked out problems, and then after a time passed on to the conscious field of the Intellect the solution of the matter. In this lesson we purpose instructing you in the methods by which this part of the Intellect may be set to work for you. Many have stumbled upon bits of this truth for themselves, and, in fact, the majority of successful men and men who have attained eminence in any walk of life have made more or less use of this truth, although they seldom understand the reason of it.

Very few Western writers have recognized the work of this plane of the mind. They have given us full and ingenious theories and examples of the workings of the Instinctive Mind, and in some cases, they have touched upon the workings and operations of the Intuitional planes, but in nearly every case they have treated the Intellect as something entirely confined to the Conscious plane of mentation. In this they have missed some of the most interesting and valuable manifestations of sub-conscious mentation.

In this lesson we will take up this particular phase of mentation, and trust to be able to point out the way to use it to the best advantage, giving some simple instructions that have been given by the Hindu teachers to their students for centuries past, such instructions of course, being modified by us to conform to the requirements and necessities of the Western student of today.

We have taken the liberty of bestowing a new title upon this phase of mentation—we have thought it well to call it "Sub-consciousing." The word "Sub," of course means "under; below;" and the word "Consciousing" is a favorite term employed by Prof. Elmer Gates, and means receiving impressions from the mind. In a general way, "Sub-consciousing," as used in this lesson, may be understood to mean "using the subconscious mind, under orders of the conscious mind."

By referring to our Eighth Lesson, we see mention made of the case of the man who indulged in "unconscious rumination," which happened to him when he read books presenting new points of view essentially opposed to his previous opinion. You will note that after days, weeks, or months, he found that to his great astonishment the old opinions were entirely rearranged, and new ones lodged there.

On the same page you will see mentioned the case of Sir William Hamilton, who discovered an important law of mathematics while walking with his wife. In this case he had been previously thinking of the missing link in his chain of reasoning, and the problem was worked out for him by the sub-conscious plane of his Intellect.

On the same page, and the one following, is found the case of Dr. Thompson, who gives an interesting account of the workings of this part of his mind, which caused him at times to experience a feeling of the uselessness of all voluntary effort, coupled with a feeling that the matter was working itself clear in his mind. He tells us that at times he seemed to be merely a passive instrument in the hands of some person other than himself, who compelled him to wait until the work was performed for him by some hidden region of the mind. When the subconscious part of the mind had completed its work, it would flash the message to his conscious mind, and he would begin to write.

On page 178 mention is also made of the great French chemist Berthelot, who relates that some of his best conceptions have flashed upon him as from the clear sky. In fact, the Eighth Lesson is largely made up of examples of this kind, and we ask the student to re-read the same, in order to refresh his mind with the truth of the workings of the sub-conscious mentality.

But you will notice in nearly all the cases mentioned, that those who related instances of the help of the sub-conscious mind had merely stumbled upon the fact that there was a part of the mind below consciousness that could and would work out problems for one, if it could somehow be set in operation. And these people trusted to luck to start that part of the mind in operation.

Or rather, they would saturate their conscious mind with a mass of material, like stuffing the stomach with food, and then bid the subconscious mind assort, separate, arrange and digest the mental food, just as does the stomach and digestive apparatus digest the natural food—outside of the realm of consciousness or volition. In none of the cases mentioned was the subconscious mind *directed* specially to perform its wonderful work. It was simply hoped that it might digest the mental material with which it had been stuffed—in pure self-defense. But there is a much better way, and we intend to tell you about it. The Hindu Yogis, or rather those who instruct their pupils in *"Raja Yoga,"* give their students directions whereby they may *direct* their sub-conscious minds to perform mental tasks for them, just as one may direct another to perform a task. They teach them the methods whereby, after having accumulated the necessary materials, they may bid the sub-conscious mentality to sort it out, rearrange, analyze, and build up from it some bit of desired knowledge. More than this, they instruct their pupils to direct and order the sub-conscious mentality to search out and report to them certain information to be found only within the mind itself—some question of philosophy or metaphysics. And when such art has been acquired, the student or Yogi rests assured that the desired result will be forthcoming in due time, and consequently dismisses the matter from his conscious mind, and busies himself with other matters, knowing that day and night, incessantly, the sub-consciousing process is going on, and that the sub-conscious mind is actively at work collecting the information, or working out the problem.

You will see at once the great superiority of this method over the old "hit-or-miss," "hope-it-will-work" plan pursued by those who have stumbled upon bits of the truth.

The Yogi teacher begins by impressing upon his students the fact that the mind is capable of extending outward toward an object, material or mental, and by examining it by methods inherent in itself, extracting knowledge regarding the object named. This is not a startling truth, because it is so common, everyone employing it more or less every day. But the process by which the knowledge is extracted is most wonderful, and really is performed below the plane of consciousness, the work of the conscious mind being chiefly concerned in *holding the Attention* upon the object. We have spoken of the importance of Attention in previous lessons, which it will be well for you to re-read, at this time.

When the student is fully impressed with the details of the process of Attention, and the subsequent unfoldment of knowledge, the Yogi proceeds to inform him that there are other means of obtaining knowledge about an object, by the employment of which the Attention may be firmly directed toward the object and then afterwards held there *unconsciously*—that is, a portion of the Attention, or a sub-conscious phase of mentation, which will hold the sub-conscious mind firmly upon the work until accomplished, leaving the conscious Attention and mentality free to employ itself with other things.

The Yogis teach the students that this new form of Attention is far more intense and powerful than is the conscious Attention, for it cannot be disturbed or shaken, or distracted from its object, and that it will work away at its task for days, months, years, or a lifetime if necessary, according to the difficulty of the task, and in fact carries its work over from one life to another, unless recalled by the Will. They teach the student that in everyone's life there is going on a greater or less degree of this sub-conscious work, carried on in obedience to a strong desire for knowledge manifested in some former life, and bearing fruit only in the present existence. Many important discoveries have been made in obedience to this law. But it is not of this phase of the matter that we wish to speak in this lesson.

The Yogi theory is that the sub-conscious intellectual faculty may be set to work under the direction of orders given by the Will. All of you know how the sub-conscious mentality will take up an order of the Will, or a strong wish, that the person be awakened at a certain hour in order to catch a train. Or, in the same way how the remembrance of a certain engagement at, say, four o'clock, will flash into the mind when the hands of the clock approach the stated hour. Nearly everyone can recall instances of this sort in his own experience.

But the Yogis go much further than this. They claim that any and all faculties of the mind may be "set going," or working on any problem, if ordered thereto by the Will. In fact, the Yogis, and their advanced students have mastered this art to such a surprising extent that they find it unnecessary to do the drudgery of thinking in the conscious field, and prefer to relegate such mental work to the sub-conscious, reserving their conscious work for the consideration of digested information and thought presented to them by the sub-conscious mind.

Their directions to their students cover a great deal of ground, and extend over a long period of time, and many of the directions are quite complicated and full of detail. But we think that we can give our students an abbreviated and condensed idea in a few pages of the lesson. And the remaining lessons of the course will also throw additional light on the subject of sub-conscious mental action, in connection with other subjects.

The Yogi takes the student when the latter is much bothered by a consideration of some knotty and perplexing philosophical subject. He bids the student relax every muscle, take the tension from every nerve—throw aside all mental strain, and then wait a few moments. Then the student is instructed to grasp the subject which he has had before his mind firmly and fixedly before his mental vision, by means of concentration. Then he is instructed to pass it on to the sub-conscious mentality by an effort of the Will, which effort is aided by forming a mental picture of the subject as a material substance, *or bundle of thought,* which is being bodily lifted up and dropped down a mental hatch-way, or trap-door, in which it sinks from sight. The student is then instructed to say to the sub-conscious mentality: "I wish this subject thoroughly analyzed, arranged, classified (and whatever else is desired) and then the results handed back to me. Attend to this."

The student is taught to speak to the sub-conscious mentality just as if it were a separate entity of being, which had been employed to do the work. He is also taught that *confident expectation* is an important part of the process, and that the degree of success depends upon the degree of this confident expectation.

In obstinate cases, the student is taught to use the Imagination freely, until he is able to make a mental image or picture of the sub-conscious mind doing what is required of it. This process clears away a mental path for the feet of the sub-conscious mind, which it will choose thereafter, as it prefers to follow the line of least resistance.

Of course, much depends upon practice—practice makes perfect, you know, in everything else, and sub-consciousing is no exception to the rule.

The student gradually acquires a proficiency in the art of sub-consciousing, and thereafter devotes his time to acquiring new facts for mental digestion, rather than bestowing it upon the mechanical act of thinking.

But a very important point to be remembered is that the Will-power back of the transferred thought-material, which Will-power is the cause of the subconscious action, depends very greatly upon the attention and interest given to the acquired material. This mass of thought-material which is to be digested, and threshed out by the sub-conscious mind, must be well saturated with interest and attention, in order to obtain the best results. In fact, interest and attention are such important aids to the Will, that any consideration of the development and acquirement of Will-power is practically a development and acquirement of attention and interest. The student is referred to previous lessons in this course in which the importance of interest and attention is explained and described.

In acquiring the mass of thought-material which is to be passed on to the sub-conscious digestion, one must concentrate a great degree of interest and attention upon each item of thought-material gathered up. The gathering of this thought-material is a matter of the greatest importance, and must not be lightly passed by. One cannot hastily gather together all sorts of thought-material, and then expect the subconscious mind to do its work properly—it will not, in fact, and the student proceeding upon any such erroneous supposition is doomed to disappointment.

The proper way to proceed, is to take up each bit of thought-material in turn, and examine it with the greatest possible interest, and consequently the greatest attention, and then after having fairly saturated it with this interested attention, place it with the pile of material which, after a while, is to be passed on to the sub-conscious mentality. Then take up the next bit of material, and after giving it similar treatment, pass it along to the pile also. Then after a while when you have gathered up the main facts of the case, proceed to consider the mass as a whole, with interest and attention, giving it as it were a "general treatment." Then drop it down the trap-door into the sub-conscious mind, with a strong command, "Attend to this thought-material," coupled with a strong expectant belief that your order will be obeyed.

The idea underlying this treatment of the thought-material with interest and attention is that by so doing a strong "Mental Image" is created, which may be easily handled by the sub-conscious mind. Remember that you are passing on "thoughts" for the sub-consciousness to act upon, and that the more tangible and real these thoughts are, the better can they be handled. Therefore, any plan that will build these thoughts up into "real" things is the plan to pursue. And attention and interest produce just this result.

If we may be pardoned for using a homely and commonplace illustration, we would say that the idea may be grasped by the illustration of boiling an egg, whereby the fluid "white" and "yolk" becomes solid and real. Also, the use of a shaving brush by a man, by which the thin lather is gradually worked up into a rich, thick, creamy mass, is an illustration. Again, the churning of butter is a favorite illustration of the Hindus, who thus call the attention of their students to the fact that thought-material if worked upon with attention and interest become "thought-forms" that may be handled by the mind just as the hands handle a material object. We ask you to think of these illustrations, for when you once grasp the idea that we wish to convey to you, you will have the secret of great thinking powers within your grasp.

And this power of sub-consciousing is not confined alone to the consideration of philosophical questions. On the contrary it is applicable to every field of human thought, and may be properly employed in any and all of them. It is useful in solving the problems of every-day life and work, as well as to the higher flights of the human mind. And we wish every one of our students to realize that in this simple lesson we are giving them the key to a great mental power.

To realize just what we are offering to you, we would remind you of the old fairy tales of all races, in which there is to be found one or more tales telling of some poor cobbler, or tailor, or carpenter, as the case may be, who had by his good deeds, gained favor with the "brownies" or good fairies, who would come each night when the man and his family were asleep, and proceed to complete the work that the artisan had laid out for the morrow. The pieces of leather would be made into shoes; the cloth would be sewed into garments; the wood would be joined, and nailed together into boxes, chairs, benches and what not. But in each case the rough materials were prepared by the artisan himself during the day.

Well, that is just what we are trying to introduce to you. A clan of mental brownies, loving and kindly disposed toward you, who are anxious and willing to help you in your work. All you have to do is to give them the proper materials, and tell then what you want done, and they will do the rest. But these mental brownies are a part of your own mentality, remember, and no alien and foreign entities, as some have imagined.

A number of people who have accidentally discovered this power of the sub-conscious mind to work out problems, and to render other valuable service to its owner, have been led to suppose that the aid really came from some other entity or intelligence. Some have thought that the messages came from friends in the spirit land, and others have believed that some high intelligence—God or his angels—was working in their behalf. Without discussing spirit communication, or Divine messages, in both of which we believe (with certain provisional reservations) we feel justified in saying that the majority of cases of this kind may be referred to the sub-conscious workings of one's own mentality.

Each of us has "a friend" in our own mind—a score of them in fact, who delight in performing services for us, if we will but allow them to do so. Not only have we a Higher Self to whom we may turn for comfort and aid in times of deep distress and necessity, but we have these invisible mental workers on the sub-conscious plane, who are very willing and glad to perform much of our mental work for us, if we will but give them the material in proper shape.

It is very difficult to impart specific directions for obtaining these results, as each case must depend to a great extent upon the peculiar circumstances surrounding it. But we may say that the main thing needed is to "lick into shape" the material, and then pass it on to the sub-conscious mind in the manner spoken of a few moments ago. Let us run over a few cases wherein this principle may be applied.

Let us suppose that you are confronted with a problem consisting of an uncertainty as to which of two or more courses to adopt in some affair of life. Each course seems to have advantages and disadvantages, and you seem unable to pass upon the matter clearly and intelligently. The more you try the more perplexed and worried do you become. Your mind seems to tire of the matter, and manifests a state which may be called "mental nausea." This state will be apparent to anyone who has had much "thinking" to do. The average person, however, persists in going over the matter, notwithstanding the tired condition of the mind, and its evident distaste for a further consideration of the subject. They will keep on forcing it back to the mind for consideration, and even at night time will keep thrashing away at the subject. Now this course is absurd. The mind recognizes that the work should be done by another part of itself—its digestive region, in fact—and naturally rebels at the finishing-up machinery being employed in work unsuited for it.

According to the Sub-consciousing plan, the best thing for the man to do would be for him first to calm and quiet his mind. Then he should arrange the main features of the problem, together with the minor details in their proper places. Then he should pass them slowly before him in review, giving a strong interest and attention to each fact and detail, as it passes before him, *but without the slightest attempt to form a decision, or come to a conclusion*. Then, having given the matter an interested and attentive review, let him *Will* that it pass on to his sub-conscious mind, forming the mental image of dropping it through the trap-door, and at the same time giving the command of the Will, "Attend to this for me!"

Then dismiss the matter from your conscious mind, by an effort of command of the Will. If you find it difficult to do this, you may soon acquire the mastery by a frequent assertion, "I have dismissed this matter from my conscious mind, and my sub-conscious mind will attend to it for me." Then, endeavor to create a mental feeling of perfect trust and confidence in the matter, and avoid all worry or anxiety about it. This may be somewhat difficult at the first trial, but will become a natural feeling after you have gained the confidence arising from successful results in several cases. The matter is one of practice, and, like anything else that is new, must be acquired by perseverance and patience. It is well worth the time and trouble, and once acquired will be regarded as something in the nature of a treasure discovered in an unexpected place. The sense of tranquility and content—of calm and confidence—that comes to one who has practiced this plan, will of itself be worth all the trouble, not to speak of the main result. To one who has acquired this method, the old worries, frettings, and general "stewed up" feeling, will seem like a relic of barbarism. The new way opens up a world of new feelings and content.

In some cases, the matter will be worked out by the sub-conscious mind in a very short time, and in fact we have known cases in which the answer would be flashed back almost instantly, almost like an inspiration. But in the majority of cases more or less time is required. The sub-conscious mind works very rapidly, but it takes time to arrange the thought-material properly, and to shape it into the desired forms. In the majority of cases, it is well to let the matter rest until the next day—a fact that gives us a clue to the old advice to "sleep over" an important proposition, before passing a final decision.

If the matter does not present itself the following day, bring it up again before the conscious mind for review. You will find that it has shaped itself up considerably, and is assuming definite form and clearness. But right here—and this is important—

do not make the mistake of again dissecting it, and meddling with it, and trying to arrange it with your conscious mind. But, instead, give it attention and interest in its new form, and then pass it back again to the sub-conscious mind for further work. You will find an improvement each time you examine it. But, right here another word of caution. Do not make the mistake of yielding to the impatience of the beginner, and keep on repeatedly bringing up the matter to see what is being done. Give it time to have the work done on it. Do not be like the boy who planted seeds, and who each day would pull them up to see whether they had sprouted, and how much.

Sooner or later, the sub-conscious mind will, of its own choice, lift up the matter and present it to you in its finished shape for the consideration of the conscious mind. The sub-conscious mind does not insist that you shall adopt its views, or accept its work, but merely hands out to you the result of its sorting, classifying and arranging. The choice and will still remain yours, but you will often find that there is seen to be one plan or path that stands out clearly from the others, and you will very likely adopt that one. The secret is that the sub-conscious mind with its wonderful patience and care has analyzed the matter, and has separated things before apparently connected. It has also found resemblances and has combined things heretofore considered opposed to each other. In short it has done for you all that you could have done with the expenditure of great work and time, and done it well. And then it lays the matter before you for your consideration and verdict.

Its whole work seems to have been in the nature of assorting, dissecting, analyzing, and arranging the evidence, and then presenting it before you in a clear, systematic shape. It does not attempt to exercise the judicial prerogative or function, but seems to recognize that its work ceases with the presentation of the edited evidence, and that of the conscious mind begins at the same point.

Now, do not confuse this work with that of the Intuition, which is a very different mental phase or plane. This sub-conscious working, just mentioned, plays an entirely different part. It is a good servant, and does not try to be more. The Intuition, on the contrary, is more like a higher friend—a friend at court, as it were, who gives us warnings and advice.

In our directions we have told you how to make use of this part of the mind, consciously and knowingly, so as to obtain the best results, and to get rid of worry and anxiety attendant upon unsettled questions. But, in fact, every one of us makes more or less use of this part of the mind unconsciously, and not realizing the important part it plays in our mental life. We are perplexed about a matter and keep it "on our minds" until we are forced to lay it aside by reason of some other demand, or when we sink to sleep. Often to our surprise we will find that when we next think of it the matter has somehow cleared up and straightened itself out, and we seem to have learned something about it that we did not know before. We do not understand it, and are apt to dismiss it as "just one of those things." In these lessons we are attempting to explain some of "those things," and to enable you to use them consciously and understandingly, instead of by chance, instinctively, and clumsily. We are teaching you Mastery of the Mind.

Now to apply the rule to another case. Suppose you wish to gather together all the information that you possess relating to a certain subject. In the first place it is certain that you know a very great deal more about any subject than you think you do. Stored away in the various recesses of the mind, or memory if you prefer that term, are stray bits of information and knowledge concerning almost any subject. But these bits of information are not associated with each other. You have never attempted to think attentively upon the particular question before you, and the facts are not correlated in the mind. It is just as if you had so many hundred pounds of anything scattered throughout the space of a large warehouse, a tiny bit here, and a tiny bit there, mixed up with thousands of other things.

You may prove this by sitting down some time and letting your thoughts run along the line of some particular subject, and you will find emerging into the field of consciousness all sorts of information that you had apparently forgotten, and each fitting itself into its proper place. Every person has had experiences of this kind. But the work of gathering together the scattered scraps of knowledge is more or less tedious for the conscious mind, and the sub-conscious mind will do the work equally well with the wear and tear on the attention. In fact, it is the sub-conscious mind that *always* does the work, even when you think it is the conscious mind. All the conscious mind does is to hold the attention firmly upon the object before it, and then let the sub-consciousness pass the material before it. But this holding the attention is tiresome work, and it is not necessary for it to expend its energies upon the details of the task, for the work may be done in an easier and simpler way.

The best way is to follow a plan similar to the one mentioned a few pages back. That is, to fix the interested attention firmly upon the question before you, until you manage to get a clear, vivid impression of *just what you want answered*. Then pass the whole matter into the sub-conscious mind with the command "Attend to this," and then leave it. Throw the whole matter off of your mind, and let the sub-conscious work go on. If possible, let the matter run along until the next morning and then take it up for consideration, when, if you have proceeded properly you will find the matter worked out, arranged in logical sequence, so that your conscious attention will be able to clearly review the string of facts, examples, illustrations, experiences, etc., relating to the matter in question.

Now, many of you will say that you would like this plan to work in cases in which you have not the time to sleep over it. In such cases we will say that it is possible to cultivate a rapid method of sub-consciousing, and in fact many business men and men of affairs have stumbled upon a similar plan, driven to the discovery by necessity. They will give a quick, comprehensive, strong flash of attention upon the subject, getting right to the heart of it, and then will let it rest in the sub-conscious mind for a moment or two, killing a minute or two of time n "preliminary conversation," until the first flash of answer comes to them.

After the first flash, and taking hold of the first loose end of the subject that presents itself to them, they will unwind a string of information and "talk" about the subject that will surprise even themselves. Many lawyers have acquired this knowledge, and are what is known as "resourceful." Such men are often confronted with questions of conditions utterly unsuspected by them a moment before. Practice has taught them the folly of fear and loss of confidence at such moments, and has also impressed upon them the truth that something within them will come to the rescue. So, presenting a confident air, they will manage to say a few platitudes or commonplaces, while the sub-conscious mind is most rapidly gathering its materials for the answer. In a moment an opening thought "flashes upon" the man, and as he continues idea after idea passes before his conscious and eager attention, sometimes so rapidly that it is almost impossible to utter them and lo! the danger is over, and a brilliant success is often snatched from the jaws of an apparent failure and defeat.

In such cases the mental demand upon the sub-conscious mind is not voiced in words, but is the result of a strong mental need. However, if one gives a quick verbal command "*Attend to this,*" the result will be heightened.

We have known of cases of men prominent in the world's affairs who made a practice of smoking a cigar during important business interviews, not because they particularly cared for tobacco, but because they had learned to appreciate the value of a moment's time for the mind to "gather itself together," as one man expressed it. A question would be asked, or a proposition advanced suddenly, demanding an immediate answer. Under the watchful eyes of the other party the questioned party tried not to show by his expression any indication of searching for an answer, for obvious reasons. So, instead, he would take a long puff at the cigar, then a slow attentive look at the ashes on its tip, and then another moment consumed in flicking the ash into the receptacle, and then came the answer, slowly, "Well, as to that—"

or some other words of that kind, prefacing the real answer which had been rapidly framed by the sub-conscious mind in time to be uttered in its proper place. The few moments of time gained had been sufficient for the sub-conscious mind to gather up its materials, and the matter to be shaped properly, without any appearance of hesitation on the part of the answerer. All of this required practice, of course, but the principle may be seen through it all and in every similar case. The point is that the man, in such cases, sets some hidden part of his mind to work for him, and when he begins to speak the matter is at least roughly "licked into shape for him."

Our students will understand, of course, that this is not advice to smoke cigars during interviews of importance, but is merely given to illustrate the principle. We have known other men to twirl a lead pencil in their fingers in a lazy sort of fashion, and then drop it at the important moment. But we must cease giving examples of this kind, lest we be accused of giving instructions in worldly wisdom, instead of teaching the use of the mind. The impressive pause of the teacher, before answering his pupil's question, is also an example of the workings of this law. One often says "stop, let me think a moment," and during his pause he does not really consciously think at all, but stares ahead in a dreamy fashion, while his sub-conscious mind does the work for him, although he little suspects the nature of the operation. One has but to look around him to realize the importance and frequent application of this truth.

And not only may the sub-conscious mind be used in the directions indicated on preceding pages, but in nearly every perplexity and problem of life may it be called upon for help. These little sub-conscious brownies are ever at our disposal, and seem to be happy to be of service to us.

And so far from being apt to get us in a position of false dependence, it is calculated to make us self-confident—for we are calling upon a part of *ourselves*, not upon some outside intelligence. If those people who never feel satisfied unless they are getting "advice" from others would only cultivate the acquaintance of this little "home adviser" within them, they would lose that dependent attitude and frame of mind, and would grow self-confident and fearless. Just imagine the confidence of one who feels that he has within him a source of knowledge equal to that of the majority of those with whom he is likely to come in contact, and he feels less afraid to face them, and look them fearlessly in the eyes. He feels that his "mind" is not confined to the little field of consciousness, but is an area infinitely greater, containing a mass of information undreamed of. Everything that the man has inherited, or brought with him from past lives—everything that he has read, heard or seen, or experienced in this life, is hidden away there in some quarter of that great sub-conscious mind, and, if he will but give the command, the "essence" of all that knowledge is his. The details may not be presented to his consciousness (often it is not, for very good occult reasons) by the result, or essence of the knowledge will pass before his attention, with sufficient examples and illustrations, or arguments to enable him to make out "a good case" for himself.

In the next lesson we will call your attention to other features and qualities of this great field of mind, showing you how you can put it to work, and Master it. Remember, always, the "I" is the Master. And its Mastery must always be remembered and asserted over all phases and planes of the mind. Do not be a slave to the sub-conscious, but be its MASTER.

MANTRAM (OR AFFIRMATION)

I have within me a great area of Mind that is under my command, and subject to my Mastery. This Mind is friendly to me, and is glad to do my bidding, and obey my orders. It will work for me when I ask it, and is constant, untiring, and faithful. Knowing this I am no longer afraid, ignorant or uninformed. The "I" is master of it all, and is asserting its authority. "I" am master over Body, Mind, Consciousness, and Sub-consciousness. I am "I"—a Centre of Power, Strength, and Knowledge. I am "I"—and "I" am Spirit, a fragment from the Divine Flame.

THE ELEVENTH LESSON

SUBCONSCIOUS CHARACTER BUILDING.

In our last lesson (the Tenth Lesson) we called your attention to the wonderful work of the sub-conscious regions of mentation in the direction of the performance of Intellectual work. Great as are the possibilities of this field of mentation in the direction named, they are equaled by the possibilities of building up character by similar methods.

Everyone realizes that one may change his character by a strenuous course of repression and training, and nearly all who read these lines have modified their characteristics somewhat by similar methods. But it is only of late years that the general public have become aware that Character might be modified, changed, and sometimes completely altered by means of an intelligent use of the sub-conscious faculties of the mind.

The word "Character" is derived from ancient terms meaning "to mark," "to engrave," etc., and some authorities inform us that the term originally arose from the word used by the Babylonian brickmakers to designate the trade mark impressed by them upon their bricks, each maker having his own mark. This is interesting, in view of the recent theories regarding the cultivation of characteristics which may be found in the current Western works on psychology. But these theories are not new to the Yogi teachers of the East, who have employed similar methods for centuries past in training their students and pupils. The Yogis have long taught that a man's character was, practically, the crude character-stuff possessed by him at his birth, modified and shaped by outside influences in the case of the ordinary man, and by deliberate self-training and shaping by the wise man. Their pupils are examined regarding their characteristics, and then directed to repress the undesirable traits, and to cultivate the desirable ones.

The Yogi practice of Character Building is based upon the knowledge of the wonderful powers of the sub-conscious plane of the mind. The pupil is not required to pursue strenuous methods of repression or cultivation, but, on the contrary, is taught that such methods are opposed to nature's plans, and that the best way is to imitate nature and to gradually unfold the desired characteristics by means of focusing the will-power and attention upon them. The weeding out of undesirable characteristics is accomplished by the pupil cultivating the characteristics directly opposed to the undesirable ones. For instance, if the pupil desires to overcome Fear, he is not instructed to concentrate on Fear with the idea of killing it out, but, instead, is taught to mentally deny that he has Fear, and then to concentrate his attention upon the ideal of Courage. When Courage is developed, Fear is found to have faded away. The positive always overpowers the negative.

In the word "ideal" is found the secret of the Yogi method of sub-conscious character building. The teachings are to the effect that "ideals" may be built up by the bestowal of attention upon them. The student is given the example of a rose bush. He is taught that the plant will grow and flourish in the measure that care and attention is bestowed upon it and *vice versa*. He is taught that the ideal of some desired characteristic is a mental rosebush, and that by careful attention it will grow and put forth leaves and flowers. He is then given some minor mental trait to develop, and is taught to dwell upon it in thought—to exercise his imagination and to mentally "see" himself attaining the desired quality. He is given mantras or affirmation to repeat, for the purpose of giving him a mental center around which to build an ideal. There is a mighty power in words, used in this way, providing that the user always thinks of the meaning of the words, and makes a mental picture of the quality expressed by them, instead of merely repeating them parrot fashion.

The Yogi student is trained gradually, until he acquires the power of conscious direction of the sub-conscious mind in the building up process, which power comes to anyone—Oriental or Occidental—who will take the trouble to practice. In fact, nearly everyone possesses and actively uses this power, although he may not be aware of it. One's character is largely the result of the quality of thoughts held in the mind, and of the mental pictures or ideals entertained by the person. The man who constantly sees and thinks of himself as unsuccessful and down-trodden is very apt to grow ideals of thought forms of these things until his whole nature is dominated by them, and his every act works toward the objectification of the thoughts. On the contrary, the man who makes an ideal of success and accomplishment finds that his whole mental nature seems to work toward that result—the objectification of the ideal.

And so, it is with every other ideal. The person who builds up a mental ideal of Jealousy will be very apt to objectify the same, and to unconsciously create condition that will give his Jealousy food upon which to feed. But this particular phase of the subject, properly belongs to our next lesson. This Eleventh Lesson is designed to point out the way by which people may mold their characters in any way they desire—supplanting undesirable characteristics by desirable ones, and developing desirable ideals into active characteristics. The mind is plastic to him who knows the secret of its manipulation.

The average person recognizes his strong and weak points of character, but is very apt to regard them as fixed and unalterable, or practically so. He thinks that he "is just as the Lord made him," and that is the end of it. He fails to recognize that his character is being unconsciously modified every day by association with others, whose suggestions are being absorbed and acted upon. And he fails to see that he is molding his own character by taking interest in certain things, and allowing his mind to dwell upon them. He does not realize that he himself is really the maker of himself, from the raw and crude material given him at his birth. He makes himself negatively or positively. Negatively, if he allows himself to be molded by the thoughts and ideals of others, and positively, if he molds himself. Everyone is doing one or the other—perhaps both. The weak man is the one who allows himself to be made by others, and the strong man is the one who takes the building process in his own hands.

The process of Character-building is so delightfully simple that its importance is apt to be overlooked by the majority of persons who are made acquainted with it. It is only by actual practice and the experiencing of results that its wonderful possibilities are borne home to one.

The Yogi student is early taught the lesson of the power and importance of character building by some strong practical example. For instance, the student is found to have certain tastes of appetite, such as a like for certain things, and a corresponding dislike for others. The Yogi teacher instructs the student in the direction of cultivating a desire and taste for the disliked thing, and a dislike for the liked thing. He teaches the student to fix his mind on the two things, but in the direction of imagining that he likes the one thing and dislikes the other. The student is taught to make a mental picture of the desired conditions, and to say, for instance, "I loathe candy—I dislike even the sight of it," and, on the other hand, "I crave tart things—I revel in the taste of them," etc., etc., at the same time trying to reproduce the taste of sweet things accompanied with a loathing, and a taste of tart things, accompanied with a feeling of delight. After a bit the student finds that his tastes are actually changing in accordance with his thoughts, and in the end, they have completely changed places. The truth of the theory is then borne home to the student, and he never forgets the lesson.

In order to reassure readers who might object to having the student left in this condition of reversed tastes, we may add that the Yogi teachers then teach him to get rid of the idea of the disliked thing, and teach him to cultivate a liking for all wholesome things, their theory being that the dislike of certain wholesome eatables has been caused by some suggestion in childhood, or by some prenatal impression, as wholesome eatables are made attractive to the taste by Nature. The idea of all this training, however, is not the cultivation of taste, but practice in mental training, and the bringing home to the student the truth of the fact that his nature is plastic to his Ego, and that it may be molded at will, by concentration and intelligent practice. The reader of this lesson may experiment upon himself along the lines of the elementary Yogi practice as above mentioned, if he so desires. He will find it possible to entirely change his dislike for certain food, etc., by the methods mentioned above. He may likewise acquire a liking for heretofore distasteful tasks and duties, which he finds it necessary to perform.

The principle underlying the whole Yogi theory of Character Building by the sub-conscious Intellect, is that the Ego is Master of the mind, and that the mind is plastic to the commands of the Ego. The Ego or "I" of the individual is the one real, permanent, changeless principle of the individual, and the mind, like the body, is constantly changing, moving, growing, and dying. Just as the body may be developed and molded by intelligent exercises, so may the mind be developed and shaped by the Ego if intelligent methods are followed.

The majority of people consider that Character is a fixed something, belonging to a man, that cannot be altered or changed. And yet they show by their everyday actions that at heart they do not believe this to be a fact, for they endeavor to change and mold the characters of those around them, by word of advice, counsel, praising or condemnation, etc.

It is not necessary to go into the matter of the consideration of the causes of character in this lesson. We will content ourselves by saying that these causes may be summed up, roughly, as follows: (1) Result of experiences in past lives; (2) Heredity; (3) Environment; (4) Suggestion from others; and (5) Auto-suggestion. But no matter how one's character has been formed, it may be modified, molded, changed, and improved by the methods set forth in this lesson, which methods are similar to what is called by Western writers, "Auto-suggestion."

The underlying idea of Auto-suggestion is the "willing" of the individual that the changes take place in his mind, the willing being aided by intelligent and tried methods of creating the new ideal or thought-form. The first requisite for the changed condition must be "desire" for the change. Unless one really desires that the change take place, he is unable to bring his Will to bear on the task. There is a very close connection between Desire and Will. Will is not usually brought to bear upon anything unless it is inspired by Desire. Some people connect the word Desire with the lower inclinations, but it is equally applicable to the higher. If one fights off a low inclination or Desire, it is because he is possessed of a higher inclination or Desire. Many Desires are really compromises between two or more conflicting Desires—a sort of average Desire, as it were.

Unless one desires to change his character, he will not make any move toward it. And in proportion to the strength of the desire, so will be the amount of will-power that is put in the task. The first thing for one to do in character building is to "want to do it." And if he finds that the "want" is not sufficiently strong to enable him to manifest the perseverance and effort necessary to bring it to a successful conclusion, then he should deliberately proceed to "build up the desire."

Desire may be built up by allowing the mind to dwell upon the subject until a desire is created. This rule works both ways, as many people have found out to their sorrow and misery. Not only may one build up a commendable desire in this way, but he may also build up a reprehensible one. A little thought will show you the truth of this statement. A young man has no desire to indulge in the excesses of a "fast" life. But after a while he hears, or reads something about others leading that sort of life, and he begins to allow his mind to dwell upon the subject, turning it around and examining it mentally, and going over it in his imagination. After a time, he begins to find a desire gradually sending forth roots and branches, and if he continues to water the thing in his imagination, before long he will find within himself a blossoming inclination, which will try to insist upon expression in action. There is a great truth behind the words of the poet:

> *"Vice is a monster of so frightful mien,*
> *That to be hated needs but to be seen.*
> *Yet seen too oft, familiar with her face,*
> *We first endure, then pity, and then embrace."*

And the follies and crimes of many a man have been due to the growing of desire within his mind, through this plan of planting the seed, and then carefully watering and tending to it—this cultivation of the growing desire. We have thought it well to give this word of warning because it will throw light upon many things that may have perplexed you, and because it may serve to call your attention to certain growing weeds of the mind that you have been nourishing.

But remember, always, that the force that leads downward may be transmuted and made to lead upward. It is just as easy to plant and grow wholesome desires as the other kind. If you are conscious of certain defects and deficiencies in your character (and who is not?) and yet find yourself not possessed of a strong enough desire to make the changes necessary, then you should commence by planting the desire seed and allowing it to grow by giving it constant care and attention. You should picture to yourself the advantages of acquiring the desirable traits of character of which you have thought. You should frequently go over and over them in your mind, imaging yourself in imagination as possessing them. You will then find that the growing desire will make headway and that you will gradually begin to "want to" possess that trait of character more and more. And when you begin to "want to" hard enough, you will find arising in your consciousness a feeling of the possession of sufficient Will-power to carry it through. Will follows the Desire. Cultivate a Desire and you will find back of it the Will to carry it through. Under the pressure of a very strong Desire men have accomplished feats akin to miracles.

If you find yourself in possession of desires that you feel are hurtful to you, you may rid yourself of them by deliberately starving them to death, and at the same time growing opposite desires. By refusing to think of the objectionable desires you refuse them the mental food upon which alone they can thrive. Just as you starve a plant by refusing it nourishing soil and water, so may you starve out an objectionable desire by refusing to give it mental food. *Remember this, for it is most important*. Refuse to allow the mind to dwell upon such desires, and resolutely turn aside the attention, *and, particularly, the imagination*, from the subject. This may call for the manifestation of a little will-power in the beginning, but it will become easier as you progress, and each victory will give you renewed strength for the next fight. But do not temporize with the desire—do not compromise with it—refuse to entertain the idea. In a fight of this kind each victory gives one added strength, and each defeat weakens one.

And while you are refusing to entertain the objectionable guest you must be sure to grow a desire of an entirely opposite nature—a desire directly opposed to the one you are starving to death. Picture the opposite desire, and think of it often. Let your mind dwell upon it lovingly and let the imagination help to build it up into form. Think of the advantages that will arise to you when you fully possess it, and let the imagination picture you as in full possession of it, and acting out your new part in life strong and vigorous in your new found power.

All this will gradually lead you to the point where you will "want to" possess this power. Then you must be ready for the next step which is "Faith" or "Confident Expectation."

Now, faith or confident expectation is not made to order in most persons, and in such cases, one must acquire it gradually. Many of you who read these lines will have an understanding of the subject that will give you this faith. But to those who lack it, we suggest that they practice on some trivial phases of the mental make-up, some petty trait of character, in which the victory will be easy and simple. From this stage they should work up to more difficult tasks, until at last they gain that faith or confident expectation that comes from persevering practice.

The greater the degree of faith or confident expectation that one carries with him in this task of character building, the greater will be his success. And this because of well-established psychological laws. Faith or confident expectation clears away the mental path and renders the work easier, while doubt or lack of faith retards the work, and acts as obstacles and stumbling blocks. Strong Desire, and Faith, or confident expectation are the first two steps. The third is Will-power.

By Will-power we do not mean that strenuous, clenching-of-fist-and-frowning-brow thing that many think of when they say "Will." Will is not manifested in this way. The true Will is called into play by one realizing the "I" part of himself and speaking the word of command from that center of power and strength. It is the voice of the "I." And it is needed in this work of character building.

So now you are ready for work, being possessed of (1) Strong Desire; (2) Faith or Confident Expectation; and (3) Will-power. With such a triple-weapon nothing but Success is possible.

Then comes the actual work. The first thing to do is to lay the track for a new Character Habit. "Habit?" you may ask in surprise. Yes, Habit! For that word gives the secret of the whole thing. Our characters are made up of inherited or acquired habits. Think over this a little and you will see the truth of it. You do certain things without a thought, because you have gotten into the habit of doing them. You act in certain ways because you have established the habit. You are in the habit of being truthful, honest, virtuous, because you have established the habit of being so. Do you doubt this? Then look around you—or look within your own heart, and you will see that you have lost some of your old habits of action, and have acquired new ones. The building up of Character is the building up of Habits. And the changing of Character is the changing of Habits. It will be well for you to settle this fact in your own mind, for it will give you the secret of many things connected with the subject.

And, remember this, that Habit is almost entirely a matter of the sub-conscious mentality. It is true that Habits originate in the conscious mind, but as they are established, they sink down into the depths of the sub-conscious mentality, and thereafter become "second nature," which, by the way, is often more powerful than the original nature of the person. The Duke of Wellington said that habit was as strong as ten natures, and he proceeded to drill habits into his army until they found it natural to act in accordance with the habits pounded into them during the drills. Darwin relates an interesting instance of the force of habit over the reason. He found that his habit of starting back at the sudden approach of danger was so firmly established that no will-power could enable him to keep his face pressed up against the cage of the cobra in the Zoological Gardens when the snake struck at him, although he knew the glass was so thick that there could be no danger, and although he exerted the full force of his will. But we venture to say that one could overcome even this strongly ingrained habit, by gradually training the sub-conscious mentality and establishing a new habit of thought and action.

It is not only during the actual process of "willing" the new habit that the work of making the new mental path goes on. In fact, the Yogis believe that the principal part of the work goes on sub-consciously between the intervals of commend, and that the real progress is made in that way, just as the real work of solving the problem is performed sub-consciously, as related in our last lesson. As an example, we may call your attention to some instances of the cultivation of physical habits. A physical task learned in the evening is much easier to perform the following-morning than it was the night before, and still easier the following Monday morning than it was on the Saturday afternoon previous.

The Germans have a saying that "we learn to skate in summer, and to swim in winter," meaning that the impression passed on to the subconscious mentality deepens and broadens during the interval of rest. The best plan is to make frequent, sharp impressions, and then to allow reasonable periods of rest in order to give the sub-conscious mentality the opportunity to do its work. By "sharp" impressions we mean impressions given under *strong attention*, as we have mentioned in some of the earlier lessons of this series.

A writer has well said: "Sow an act, reap a habit; sow a habit, reap a character; sow a character, reap a destiny," thus recognizing habit as the source of character. We recognize this truth in our training of children, forming goods habits of character by constant repetition, by watchfulness, etc. Habit acts as a *motive* when established, so that while we think we are acting without motive we may be acting under the strong motive power of some well-established habit. Herbert Spencer has well said: "The habitually honest man does what is right, not consciously because he 'ought' but with simple satisfaction; and is ill at ease till it is done."

Some may object that this idea of Habit as a basis of Character may do away with the idea of a developed moral conscientiousness, as for instance, Josiah Royce who says: "The establishment of organized habit is never in itself enough to ensure the growth of an enlightened moral conscientiousness" but to such we would say that one must "want to" cultivate a high character before he will create the habits usual to the same, and the "want to" is the sign of the "moral conscientiousness," rather than the habit. And the same is true of the "ought to" side of the subject. The "ought to" arises in the conscious mind in the beginning, and inspires the cultivation of the habit, although the latter after a while becomes automatic, a matter of the sub-conscious mentality, without any "ought to" attachment. It then becomes a matter of "like to."

Thus, we see that the molding, modifying, changing, and building of Character is largely a matter of the establishing of Habits. And what is the best way to establish Habits? becomes our next question. The answer of the Yogi is: "Establish a Mental Image, and then build your Habit around it." And in that sentence, he has condensed a whole system.

Everything we see having a form is built around a mental image—either the mental image of some man, some animal, or of the Absolute. This is the rule of the universe, and in the matter of character-building we but follow a well-established rule. When we wish to build a house, we first think of "house" in a general way. Then we begin to think of "what kind" of a house. Then we go into details. Then we consult an architect, and he makes us a plan, which plan is his mental image, suggested by our mental image. Then, the plan once decided upon, we consult the builder, and at last the house stands completed—an objectified Mental Image. And so, it is with every created thing—all manifestation of a Mental Image.

And so, when we wish to establish a trait of Character, we must form a clear, distinct Mental Image of what we wish to be. This is an important step. Make your picture clear and distinct, and fasten it in your mind. Then begin to build around it. Let your thoughts dwell upon the mental picture. Let your imagination see yourself as possessed of the desired trait, and *acting it out*. Act it out in your imagination, over and over again, as often as possible, persevering, and continuously, seeing yourself manifesting the trait under a variety of circumstances and conditions. As you continue to do this you will find that you will gradually begin to express the thought in action—to objectify the subjective mental image. It will become "natural" for you to act more and more in accordance with your mental image, until at last the new habit will become firmly fixed in your mind, and will become your natural mode of action and expression.

This is no vague, visionary theory. It is a well-known and proven psychological fact, and thousands have worked marvelous changes in their character by its means.

Not only may one elevate his moral character in this way, but he may mold his "work-a-day" self to better conform to the needs of his environment and occupation. If one lacks Perseverance, he may attain it; if one is filled with Fear, he may supplant it with Fearlessness; if one lacks Self-confidence, he may gain it. In fact, there is no trait that may not be developed in this way. People have literally "made themselves over" by following this method of character-building. The great trouble with the race has been that persons have not realized that they *could* do these things. They have thought that they were doomed to remain just the creatures that they found themselves to be. They did not realize that the work of creation was not ended, and that they had within themselves a creative power adapted to the needs of their case. When man first realizes this truth, and proves it by practice, he becomes another being. He finds himself superior to environment, and training—he finds that he may ride over these things. He makes *his own environment*, and *he trains himself*.

In some of the larger schools in England and the United States, certain scholars who have developed and manifested the ability to control themselves and their actions are placed on the role of a grade called the "Self-governed grade." Those in this grade act as if they had memorized the following words of Herbert Spencer: "In the supremacy of self-control consists one of the perfections of the ideal man. Not to be impulsive—not to be spurred hither and thither by each desire—but to be self-restrained, self-balanced, governed by the just decision of the feelings in council assembled * * * that it is which moral education strives to produce." And this is the desire of the writer of this lesson—to place each student in the "Self-governed class."

We cannot attempt, in the short space of a single lesson, to map out a course of instruction in Character Building adapted to the special needs of each individual. But we think that what we have said on the subject should be sufficient to point out the method for each student to map out a course for himself, following the general rules given above. As a help to the student, however, we will give a brief course of instruction for the cultivation of one desirable trait of character. The general plan of this course may be adapted to fit the requirements of *any other case*, if intelligence is used by the student. The case we have selected is that of a student who has been suffering from "a lack of Moral Courage—a lack of Self-Confidence—an inability to maintain my poise in the presence of other people—an inability to say 'No!'—a feeling of Inferiority to those with whom I come in contact." The brief outline of the course of practice given in this case is herewith given:

PRELIMINARY THOUGHT. You should fix firmly in your mind the fact that you are the Equal of any and every man. You come from the same source. You are an expression of the same One Life. In the eyes of the Absolute you are the equal of any man, even the highest in the land. Truth is "Things as God sees them"—and in Truth you and the man are equal, and, at the last, One. All feelings of Inferiority are illusions, errors, and lies, and have no existence in Truth. When in the company of others remember this fact and realize that the Life Principle in you is talking to the Life Principle in them. Let the Life Principle flow through you, and endeavor to forget your personal self. At the same time, endeavor to see that same Life Principle, behind and beyond the personality of the person in whose presence you are. He is by a personality hiding the Life Principle, just as you are. Nothing more—nothing less! You are both One in Truth. Let the conscious of the "I" beam forth and you will experience an uplift and sense of Courage, and the other will likewise feel it. You have within you the Source of Courage, Moral and Physical, and you have naught to Fear—Fearlessness is your Divine Heritage, avail yourself of it.

You have Self-Conscience, for the Self is the "I" within you, not the petty personality, and you must have confidence in that "I." Retreat within yourself until you feel the presence of the "I," and then will you have a Self-Confidence that nothing can shake or disturb. Once having attained the permanent consciousness of the "I," you will have poise. Once having realized that you are a Center of Power, you will have no difficulty in saying "No!" when it is right to do so. Once having realized your true nature—your Real Self—you will lose all sense of Inferiority, and will know that you are a manifestation of the One Life and have behind you the strength, power, and grandeur of the Cosmos. Begin by realizing YOURSELF, and then proceed with the following methods of training the mind.

WORD IMAGES. It is difficult for the mind to build itself around an idea, unless that idea be expressed in words. A word is the center of an idea, just as the idea is the center of the mental image, and the mental image the center of the growing mental habit. Therefore, the Yogis always lay great stress upon the use of words in this way. In the particular case before us, we should suggest the holding before you of a few words crystallizing the main thought.

We suggest the words "I Am"; Courage; Confidence; Poise; Firmness; Equality. Commit these words to memory, and then endeavor to fix in your mind a clear conception of the meaning of each word, so that each may stand for a Live Idea when you say it. Beware of parrot-like or phonographic repetition. Let each word's meaning stand out clearly before you, so that when you repeat it you may *feel* its meaning. Repeat the words over frequently, when opportunity presents itself, and you will soon begin to notice that they act as a strong mental tonic upon you, producing a bracing, energizing effect. And each time you repeat the words, understandingly, you have done something to clear away the mental path over which you wish to travel.

PRACTICE

When you are at leisure, and are able to indulge in "day dreams" without injury to your affairs of life, call your imagination into play and endeavor to picture yourself as being possessed of the qualities indicated by the words named. Picture yourself under the most trying circumstances, making use of the desired qualities, and manifesting them fully. Endeavor to picture yourself as acting out your part well, and exhibiting the desired qualities. Do not be ashamed to indulge in these day-dreams, for they are the prophecies of the things to follow, and you are but rehearsing your part before the day of the performance.

Practice makes perfect, and if you accustom yourself to acting in a certain way in imagination, you will find it much easier to play your part when the real performance occurs. This may seem childish to many of you, but if you have an actor among your acquaintances, consult him about it, and you will find that he will heartily recommend it. He will tell you what practice does for one in this direction, and how repeated practice and rehearsals may fix a character so firmly in a man's mind that he may find it difficult to divest himself of it after a time. Choose well the part you wish to play—the character you wish to be yours—and then after fixing it well in your mind, practice, practice, practice. Keep your ideal constantly before you, and endeavor to grow into it. And you will succeed, if you exercise patience and perseverance.

But, more than this. Do not confine your practice to mere private rehearsal. You need some "dress rehearsals" as well—rehearsals in public. Therefore, after you get well started in your work, manage to exercise your growing character-habits in your everyday life. Pick out the little cases first and "try it on them."

You will find that you will be able to overcome conditions that formerly bothered you much. You will become conscious of a growing strength and power coming from within, and you will recognize that you are indeed a changed person. Let your thought express itself in action, whenever you get a good chance. But do not try to force chances just to try your strength. Do not, for instance, try to force people to ask for favors that you may say "No!" You will find plenty of genuine tests without forcing any. Accustom yourself to looking people in the eye, and feeling the power that is back of you, and within you.

You will soon be able to see through their personality, and realize that it is just one portion of the One Life gazing at another portion, and that therefore there is nothing to be afraid of. A realization of your Real Self will enable you to maintain your poise under trying circumstances, if you will but throw aside your false idea about your personality. Forget yourself—your little personal self—for a while, and fix your mind on the Universal Self of which you are a part. All these things that have worried you are but incidents of the Personal Life, and are seen to be illusions when viewed from the standpoint of the Universal Life.

Carry the Universal Life with you as much as possible into your everyday life. It belongs there as much as anywhere, and will prove to be a tower of strength and refuge to you in the perplexing situations of your busy life.

Remember always that the Ego is master of the mental states and habits, and that the Will is the direct instrument of the Ego, and is always ready for its use. Let your soul be filled with the strong Desire to cultivate those mental habits that will make you Strong. Nature's plan is to produce Strong Individual expressions of herself, and she will be glad to give you her aid in becoming strong. The man who wishes to strengthen himself will always find great forces back of him to aid him in the work, for is he not carrying out one of Nature's pet plans, and one which she has been striving for throughout the ages.

Anything that tends to make you realize and express your Mastery, tends to strengthen you, and places at your disposal Nature's aid. You may witness this in everyday life—Nature seems to like *strong* individuals, and delights in pushing them ahead. By Mastery, we mean mastery over your own lower nature, as well as over outside nature, of course. The "I" is Master—forget it not, O student, and assert it constantly. Peace be with you.

MANTRAM (OR AFFIRMATION)

I am the Master of my Mental Habits—I control my Character. I Will to be Strong, and summon the forces of my Nature to my aid.

THE TWELFTH LESSON

SUB-CONSCIOUS INFLUENCES.

In this lesson we wish to touch upon a certain feature of sub-conscious mentation that has been much dwelt upon by certain schools of western writers and students during the past twenty years, but which has also been misunderstood, and, alas, too often misused, by some of those who have been attracted to the subject. We allude to what has been called the "Power of Thought."

While this power is very real, and like any other of the forces of nature may be properly used and applied in our everyday life, still many students of the power of the Mind have misused it and have stooped to practices worthy only of the followers of the schools of "Black Magic." We hear on all sides of the use of "treatments" for selfish and often base ends, those following these practices seeming to be in utter ignorance of the occult laws brought into operation, and the terrible reaction inevitably falling to the lot of those practicing this negative form of mental influence. We have been amazed at the prevailing ignorance concerning the nature and effects of this improper use of mental force, and at the same time, at the common custom of such selfish, improper uses. This, more particularly, when the true occultist knows that these things are not necessary, even to those who seek "Success" by mental forces. There is a true method of the use of mental forces, as well as an improper use, and we trust that in this lesson we may be able to bring the matter sharply and clearly before the minds of our students.

In our first course (The Fourteen Lessons) in the several lessons entitled, respectively, "Thought Dynamics," "Telepathy, etc.," and "Psychic Influence," we have given a general idea of the effect of one mind upon other minds, and many other writers have called the attention of the Western world to the same facts. There has been a general awakening of interest in this phase of the subject among the Western people of late years, and many and wonderful are the theories that have been advanced among the conflicting schools regarding the matter. But, notwithstanding the conflicting theories, there is a general agreement upon the fundamental facts. They all agree that the mental forces may be used to affect oneself and others, and many have started in to use these mental forces for their own selfish ends and purposes, believing that they were fully justified in so doing, and being unaware of the web of psychic causes and effects which they were weaving around them by their practices.

Now, at the beginning, let us impress upon the minds of our students the fact that while it is undoubtedly true that people who are unaware of the true sources of strength within them, may be, and often are affected by mental force exerted by others, it is equally true that no one can be adversely affected in this way providing he realizes the "I" within himself, which is the only Real part of him, and which is an impregnable tower of strength against the assaults of others. There is no cause for all of this fear that is being manifested by many Western students of thought-power, who are in constant dread of being "treated" adversely by other people. The man or woman who realizes the "I" within, may by the slightest exercise of the Will surround himself with a mental aura which will repel adverse thought-waves emanating from the minds of others. Nay, more than this—the habitual recognition of the "I," and a few moments' meditation upon it each day, will of itself erect such an aura, and will charge this aura with a vitality that will turn back adverse thought, and cause it to return to the source from which it came, where it will serve the good purpose of bringing to the mistaken mind originating it, the conviction that such practices are hurtful and to be avoided.

This realization of the "I," which we brought out in the first few lessons of the present series, is the best and only real method of self-protection. This may be easily understood, when we remind you that the whole phenomena of mental influencing belong to the "illusion" side of existence—the negative side—and that the Real and Positive side must of necessity be stronger. Nothing can affect the Real in you—and the nearer you get to the Real, in realization and understanding, the stronger do you become. *This is the whole secret*. Think it over.

But there are comparatively few people who are able to rest firmly in the "I" consciousness all the time and the others demand help while they are growing. To such, we would say "Creep as close the Realization of the I, as possible, and rest your spiritual feet firmly upon the rock of the Real Self." If you feel that people, circumstances, or things are influencing you unduly, stand up boldly, and deny the influence. Say something like this, "I DENY the power or influence of persons, circumstances, or things to adversely affect me. I ASSERT my Reality, Power and Dominion over these things."

These words may seem very simple, but when uttered with the consciousness of the Truth underlying them, they become as a mighty force. You will understand, of course, that there is no magic or virtue in the words themselves—that is, in the grouping of the letters forming the words, or the sounds of the words—the virtue resting in the *idea* of which the words are the expression. You will be surprised at the effect of this STATEMENT upon depressing, or adverse influences surrounding you. If you—*you* who are reading these words now—feel yourself subject to any adverse or depressing influences, will then stand up erect, throwing your shoulders back, raising your head, and looking boldly and fearlessly ahead, and repeat these words firmly, and with faith, you will feel the adverse influences disappearing. You will almost see the clouds falling back from you. Try it now, before reading further, and you will become conscious of a new strength and power.

You are perfectly justified in thus denying adverse influence. You have a perfect right to drive back threatening or depressing thought-clouds. You have a perfect right to take your stand upon the Rock of Truth—your Real Self—and demand your Freedom. These negative thoughts of the world in general, and of some people in particular, belong to the dark side of life, and you have a right to demand freedom from them. You do not belong to the same idea of life, and it is your privilege—yes, your duty—to repel them and bid them disappear from your horizon. You are a Child of Light, and it is your right and duty to assert your freedom from the things of darkness.

You are merely asserting the Truth when you affirm your superiority and dominion over these dark forces. And in the measure of your Recognition and Faith, will be the power at your disposal. Faith and Recognition renders man a god. If we could but fully recognize and realize just what we are, we could rise above this entire plane of negative, dark world of thought. But we have become so blinded and stupefied with the race-thought of fear and weakness, and so hypnotized with the suggestions of weakness that we hear on all sides of us, that even the best of us find it hard to avoid occasionally sinking back into the lower depths of despair and discouragement. But, let us remember this, brothers and sisters, that these periods of "back-sliding" become less frequent, and last a shorter time, as we proceed. Bye-and-bye we shall escape them altogether.

Some may think that we are laying too much stress upon the negative side of the question, but we feel that what we have said is timely, and much needed by many who read these lessons. There has been so much said regarding this negative, adverse power of thought, that it is well that all should be taught that it is in their power to rise above this thing— that the weapon for its defeat is already in their hand.

The most advanced student may occasionally forget that he is superior to the adverse influence of the race-thought, and other clouds of thought influence that happen to be in his neighborhood. When we think of how few there are who are sending forth the positive, hopeful, thought-waves, and how many are sending forth continually the thoughts of discouragement, fear, and despair, it is no wonder that at times there comes to us a feeling of discouragement, helplessness, and "what's the use." But we must be ever alert, to stand up and *deny these things out of existence* so far as our personal thought world is concerned. There is a wonderful occult truth in the last sentence. We are the makers, preservers, and destroyers of our personal thought-world.

We may bring into it that which we desire to appear; we may keep there what we wish, cultivating, developing and unfolding the thought-forms that we desire; we may destroy that which we wish to keep out. The "I" is the master of its thought-world. Think over this great truth, O student! By Desire we call into existence—by affirmation we preserve and encourage—by Denial we destroy. The Hindus in their popular religious conceptions picture the One Being as a Trinity, composed of Brahma, the Creator; Vishnu, the Preserver, and Siva, the Destroyer—not three gods, as is commonly supposed, but a Trinity composed of three aspects of Deity or Being. This idea of the threefold Being is also applicable to the Individual—"as above so below." The "I" is the Being of the Individual, and the thought-world is its manifestation. It creates, preserves, and destroys—as it Will. Carry this idea with you, and realize that your individual thought-world is your own field of manifestation. In it you are constantly creating—constantly preserving—constantly destroying. And if you can destroy anything in your own thought-world you remove it from its field of activity, so far as you are concerned.

And if you create anything in your own thought-world, you bring it into active being, so far as you are concerned. And if you preserve anything, you keep it by you in effect and full operation and influence in your life. This truth belongs to the higher phases of the subject, for its explanation is inextricably bound up in the explanation of the "Thing-in-Itself"—the Absolute and Its Manifestations. But even what we have said above, should give to the alert student sufficient notice to cause him to grasp the facts of the case, and to apply the principles in his own life.

If one lives on the plane of the race-thought, he is subject to its laws, for the law of cause and effect is in full operation on each plane of life. But when one raises himself above the race-thought, and on to the plane of the Recognition of the Real Self—The "I"—then does he extricate himself from the lower laws of cause and effect, and places himself on a higher plane of causation, in which he plays a much higher part. And so, we are constantly reminding you that your tower of strength and refuge lies on the higher plane. But, nevertheless, we must deal with the things and laws of the lower plane, because very few who read these lessons are able to rest entirely upon the higher plane. The great majority of them have done no more than to lift themselves partially on to the higher plane, and they are consequently living on both planes, partly in each, the consequence being that there is a struggle between the conflicting laws of the two planes. The present stage is one of the hardest on the Path of Attainment, and resembles the birth-pains of the physical body. But you are being born into a higher plane, and the pain after becoming the most acute will begin to ease, and in the end will disappear, and then will come peace and calm. When the pain becomes the most acute, then be cheered with the certainty that you have reached the crisis of your new spiritual birth, and that you will soon gain peace.

And then you will see that the peace and bliss will be worth all the pain and struggle. Be brave, fellow followers of The Path—Deliverance is nigh. Soon will come the Silence that follows the Storm. The pain that you are experiencing—ah, well do we know that you are experiencing the pain—is not punishment, but is a necessary part of your growth. All Life follows this plan—the pains of labor and birth ever precede the Deliverance. Such is Life—and Life is based upon Truth—and all is well with the world. We did not intend to speak of these things in this lesson, but as we write there comes to us a great cry for help and a word of encouragement and hope, from the Class which is taking this course of lessons, and we feel bound to respond as we have done. Peace be with you—one and all.

And, now we will begin our consideration of the laws governing what we have called "Sub-conscious Influence."

All students of the Occult are aware of the fact that men may be, and are, largely influenced by the thoughts of others. Not only is this the case in instances where thoughts are directed from the mind of one person to the mind of another, but also when there is no special direction or intention in the thought sent forth. The vibrations of thoughts linger in the astral atmosphere long after the effort that sent forth the thought has passed. The astral atmosphere is charged with the vibrations of thinkers of many years past, and still possesses sufficient vitality to affect those whose minds are ready to receive them at this time. And we all attract to us thought vibrations corresponding in nature with those which we are in the habit of entertaining. The Law of Attraction is in full operation, and one who makes a study of the subject may see instances of it on all sides.

We invite to ourselves these thought vibrations by maintaining and entertaining thoughts along certain lines. If we cultivate a habit of thinking along the lines of Cheerfulness, Brightness and Optimism, we attract to ourselves similar thought vibrations of others and we will find that before long we will find all sorts of cheerful thoughts pouring into our minds from all directions. And, likewise, if we harbor thoughts of Gloom, Despair, Pessimism, we lay ourselves open to the influx of similar thoughts which have emanated from the minds of others. Thoughts of Anger, Hate, or Jealousy attract similar thoughts which serve to feed the flame and keep alive the fire of these low emotions. Thoughts of Love tend to draw to ourselves the loving thoughts of others which tend to fill us with a glow of loving emotion.

And not only are we affected in this way by the thoughts of others, but what is known as "Suggestion" also plays an important part in this matter of sub-conscious influence. We find that the mind has a tendency to reproduce the emotions, moods, shades of thought, and feelings of other persons, as evidenced by their attitude, appearance, facial expression, or words.

If we associate with persons of a gloomy temperament, we run the risk of "catching" their mental trouble by the law of suggestion, unless we understand this law and counteract it. In the same way we find that cheerfulness is contagious, and if we keep in the company of cheerful people, we are very apt to take on their mental quality. The same rule applies to frequenting the company of unsuccessful or successful people, as the case may be. If we allow ourselves to take up the suggestions constantly emanating from them, we will find that our minds will begin to reproduce the tones, attitudes, characteristics, dispositions and traits of the other persons, and before long we will be living on the same mental plane. As we have repeatedly said, these things are true only when we allow ourselves to "take on" the impressions, but unless one has mastered the law of suggestion, and understands its principles and operations he is more or less apt to be affected by it.

All of you readily recall the effect of certain persons upon others with whom they come in contact. One has a faculty of inspiring with vigor and energy those in whose company he happens to be. Another depresses those around him, and is avoided as a "human wet-blanket." Another will cause a feeling of uneasiness in those around him, by reason of his prevailing attitude of distrust, suspicion, and low cunning. Some carry an atmosphere of health around them, while others seem to be surrounded with a sickly aura of disease, even when their physical condition does not seem to indicate the lack of health. Mental states have a subtle way of impressing themselves upon us, and the student who will take the trouble to closely observe those with whom he comes in contact will receive a liberal education along these lines.

There is of course a great difference in the degree of suggestibility among different persons. There are those who are almost immune, while at the other end of the line are to be found others who are so constantly and strongly impressed by the suggestions of others, conscious or unconscious, that they may be said to scarcely have any independent thought or will of their own. But nearly all persons are suggestible to a greater or lesser degree.

It must not be supposed from what we have said that all suggestions are "bad," harmful, or undesirable. Many suggestions are very good for us, and coming at the right time have aided us much. But, nevertheless, it is well to always *let your own mind pass upon* these suggestions, before allowing them to manifest in your sub-conscious mind. Let the final decision be your own—and not the will of another—although you may have considered outside suggestions in connection with the matter.

Remember always that YOU are an Individual, having a mind and Will of your own. Rest firmly upon the base of your "I" consciousness, and you will find yourself able to manifest a wonderful strength against the adverse suggestions of others. Be your own Suggestor—train and influence your sub-conscious mind Yourself, and do not allow it to be tampered with by the suggestions of others. Grow the sense of Individuality.

There has been much written of recent years in the Western world regarding the effect of the Mental Attitude upon Success and attainment upon the material plane. While much of this is nothing but the wildest imagining, still there remains a very firm and solid substratum of truth underlying it all.

It is undoubtedly true that one's prevailing mental attitude is constantly manifesting and objectifying itself in his life. Things, circumstances, people, plans, all seem to fit into the general ideal of the strong mental attitude of a man. And this from the operation of mental law along a number of lines of action.

In the first place, the mind when directed toward a certain set of objects becomes very alert to discover things concerning those objects—to seize upon things, opportunities, persons, ideas, and facts tending to promote the objects thought of. The man who is looking for facts to prove certain theories, invariably finds them, and is also quite likely to overlook facts tending to disprove his theory. The Optimist and the Pessimist passing along the same streets, each sees thousands of examples tending to fit in with his idea. As Kay says: "When one is engaged in seeking for a thing, if he keeps the image of it clearly before the mind, he will be very likely to find it, and that too, probably, where it would otherwise have escaped his notice.

So, when one is engaged in thinking on a subject, thoughts of things resembling it, or bearing upon it, and tending to illustrate it, come up on every side. Truly, we may well say of the mind, as has been said of the eye, that 'it perceives only what it brings within the power of perceiving.'" John Burroughs has well said regarding this that "No one ever found the walking fern who did not have the walking fern in his mind. A person whose eye is full of Indian relics picks them up in every field he walks through. They are quickly recognized because the eye has been commissioned to find them."

When the mind is kept firmly fixed upon some ideal or aim, its whole and varied powers are bent toward the realization and manifestation of that ideal. In thousands of ways the mind will operate to objectify the subjective mental attitude, a great proportion of the mental effort being accomplished along sub-conscious lines. It is of the greatest importance to one who wishes to succeed in any undertaking, to keep before his mind's eye a clear mental image of that which he desires. He should picture the thing desired, and himself as securing it, until it becomes almost real. In this way he calls to his aid his entire mental force and power, along the sub-conscious lines, and, as it were, makes a clear path over which he may walk to accomplishment.

Bain says regarding this: "By aiming at a new construction, we must clearly conceive what is aimed at. Where we have a very distinct and intelligible model before us, we are in a fair way to succeed; in proportion as the ideal is dim and wavering, we stagger or miscarry." Maudsley says: "We cannot do an act voluntarily unless we know what we are going to do, and we cannot know exactly what we are going to do until we have taught ourselves to do it." Carpenter says: "The continued concentration of attention upon a certain idea gives it a dominant power, not only over the mind, but over the body." Muller says: "The idea of our own strength gives strength to our movements. A person who is confident of effecting anything by muscular efforts will do it more easily than one not so confident of his own power." Tanner says: "To believe firmly is almost tantamount in the end to accomplishment. Extraordinary instances are related showing the influence of the will over even the involuntary muscles."

Along the same lines, many Western writers have added their testimony to the Yogi principle of the manifestation of thought into action. Kay has written: "A clear and accurate idea of what we wish to do, and how it is to be effected, is of the utmost value and importance in all the affairs of life. A man's conduct naturally shapes itself according to the ideas in his mind, and nothing contributes more to success in life than having a high ideal and keeping it constantly in view. Where such is the case one can hardly fail in attaining it. Numerous unexpected circumstances will be found to conspire to bring it about, and even what seemed at first to be hostile may be converted into means for its furtherance; while by having it constantly before the mind he will be ever ready to take advantage of any favoring circumstances that may present themselves." Along the same lines, Foster has written these remarkable words: "It is wonderful how even the casualties of life seem to bow to a spirit that will not bow to them, and yield to subserve a design which they may, in their first apparent tendency, threaten to frustrate. When a firm, decisive spirit is recognized, it is curious to see how the space clears around a man and leaves him room and freedom." Simpson has said: "A passionate desire and an unwearied will can perform impossibilities, or what seem to be such to the cold and feeble." And Maudsley gives to aspiring youth a great truth, when he says: "Thus it is that aspirations are often prophecies, the harbingers of what a man shall be in a condition to perform." And we may conclude the paragraph by quoting Lytton: "Dream, O youth, dream manfully and nobly, and thy dreams shall be prophets."

This principle of the power of the Mental Image is strongly impressed upon the mind of the *chela*, or student, by the Yogi teachers. The student is taught that just as the house is erected in accordance with the plan of the architect, so is one's life built in accordance with the prevailing Mental Image.

The mind sub-consciously molds itself around the prevailing mental image or attitude, and then proceeds to draw upon the outer world for material with which to build in accordance with the plan. Not only is one's character built in this way, but the circumstances and incidents of his life follow the same rule. The Yogi student is instructed into the mysteries of the power of the mind in this direction, not that he may make use of it to build up material success, or to realize his personal desires—for he is taught to avoid these things—but he is fully instructed, nevertheless, that he may understand the workings of the law around him.

And it is a fact well known to close students of the occult, that the few who have attained extraordinarily high degrees of development, make use of this power in order to help the race. Many a world movement has been directed by the mind, or minds, of some of these advanced souls who were able to see the ideal of evolution ahead of the race, and by visualizing the same, and concentrating upon it in meditation, actually hastened the progress of the evolutionary wave, and caused to actually manifest that which they saw, and upon which they had meditated.

It is true that some occultists have used similar plans to further their own selfish personal ends—often without fully realizing just what power they were employing—but this merely illustrates the old fact that the forces of Nature may be used rightly and wrongly. And it is all the more reason why those who are desirous of advancing the race—of assisting in the evolution of the world—should make use of this mighty power in their work. Success is not reprehensible, notwithstanding the fact that many have interpreted and applied the word in such a matter as to make it appear as if it had no other meaning or application other than the crude, material selfish one generally attributed to it, by reason of its misuse. The Western world is playing its part in the evolution of the race, and its keynote is "Accomplishment." Those who have advanced so high that they are able to view the world of men, as one sees a valley from a mountain peak, recognize what this strenuous Western life means. They see mighty forces in operation—mighty principles being worked out by those who little dream of the ultimate significance of that which they are doing.

Mighty things are before the Western world to-day—wonderful changes are going on—great things are in the womb of time, and the hour of birth draws near. The men and women in the Western world feel within them the mighty urge to "accomplish" something—to take an active part in the great drama of life. And they are right in giving full expression to this urge, and are doing well in using every legitimate means in the line of expression. And this idea of the Mental Attitude, or the Mental Image, is one of the greatest factors in this striving for Success.

In this lesson we do not purpose giving "Success Talks" for our students. These lessons are intended to fill another field, and there are many other channels of information along the lines named. What we wish to do is to point out to our students the meaning of all this strenuous striving of the age, in the Western world, and the leading principle employed therein. The great achievements of the material world are being accomplished by means of the Power of the Mind. Men are beginning to understand that "Thought manifests itself in Action," and that Thought attracts to itself the things, persons and circumstances in harmony with itself. The Power of Mind is becoming manifest in hundreds of ways.

The power of Desire, backed by Faith and Will, is beginning to be recognized as one of the greatest of known dynamic forces. The life of the race is entering into a new and strange stage of development and evolution, and in the years to come MIND will be seen, more clearly and still more clearly, to be the great principle underlying the world of material things and happenings. That "All is Mind" is more than a dreamy, metaphysical utterance, is being recognized by the leaders in the world's thought.

As we have said, great changes are before the world and the race, and every year brings us nearer to the beginning of them. In fact, the beginning is already upon us. Let any thinker stop and reflect over the wonderful changes of the past six years—since the dawning of the Twentieth Century, and he will be dull indeed if he sees not the trend of affairs. We are entering into a new Great Cycle of the race, and the old is being prepared for being dropped off like an old worn-out husk. Old conventions, ideals, customs, laws, ethics, and things sociological, economical, theological, philosophical, and metaphysical have been outgrown, and are about to be "shed" by the race. The great cauldron of human thought is bubbling away fiercely, and many things are rising to its surface. Like all great changes, the good will come only with much pain—all birth is with pain. The race feels the pain and perpetual unrest, but knows not what is the disease nor the remedy. Many false cases of diagnosis and prescription are even now noticeable, and will become still more in evidence as the years roll by. Many self-styled saviors of the race—prescribers for the pain of the soul and mind—will arise and fall. But out of it all will come that for which the race now waits.

The changes that are before us are as great as the changes in thought and life described in the late novel by H. G. Wells, entitled "*In the Days of the Comet*." In fact, Mr. Wells has indicated in that story some of the very changes that the advanced souls of the race have informed their students are before the race—the prophetic insight of the writer named seems marvelous, until one realizes that even that writer is being used as a part of the mental machinery of The Change itself. But the change will not come about by reason of the new gas caused by the brushing of the earth's surface by a passing comet. It will come from the unfolding of the race mind, the process being now under way. Are not the signs of mental unrest and discomfort becoming more and more apparent as the days go by?

The pain is growing greater, and the race is beginning to fret and chafe, and moan. It knows not what it wants, but it knows that it feels pain and wants something to relieve that pain. The old things are beginning to totter and fall, and ideas rendered sacred by years of observance are being brushed aside with a startling display of irreverence. Under the surface of our civilization, we may hear the straining and groaning of the ideas and principles that are striving to force their way out on to the plane of manifestation.

Men are running hither and thither crying for a leader and a savior. They are trying this thing, and that thing, but they find not that which they seek. They cry for Satisfaction, but it eludes them. And yet all this search and disappointment is part of the Great Change, and is preparing the race for That-which-must-Come. And yet the relief will not come from any Thing or Things. It will come from Within. Just as when, in Well's story, things righted themselves when the vapor of the comet had cleared men's minds, so will Things take their new places when the mind of the race becomes cleared by the new unfoldment that is even now under way.

Men are beginning to feel each other's pains—they find themselves unsatisfied by the old rule of "every man for himself, and the devil take the hindmost"—it used to content the successful, but now it doesn't seem to be so satisfying. The man on top is becoming lonesome, and dissatisfied, and discontented—his success seems to appall him, in some mysterious manner. And the man underneath feels stirring within himself strange longings and desires, and dissatisfaction. And new frictions are arising, and new and startling ideas are being suddenly advanced, supported and opposed.

And the relations between people seem to be unsatisfactory. The old rules, laws, and bonds are proving irksome. New, strange, and wild thoughts are coming into the minds of people, which they dare not utter to their friends—and yet these same friends are finding similar ideas within themselves. And somehow, underneath it all is to be found a certain Honesty—yes, there is where the trouble seems to come, *the world is tiring of hypocrisy and dishonesty in all human relations*, and is crying aloud to be led back, someway, to Truth and Honesty in Thought and Action. But it does not see the way out! And it will not see the way out, until the race-mind unfolds still further. And the pain of the new unfoldment is stirring the race to its depths. From the deep recesses of the race-mind are rising to the surface old passions, relics from the cave-dweller days, and all sorts of ugly mental relics of the past. And they will continue to rise and show themselves until at last the bubbling pot will begin to quiet down, and then will come a new peace, and the best will come to the surface—the essence of all the experiences of the race.

To our students, we would say: During the struggle ahead of the race, play well your part, doing the best you can, living each day by itself, meeting each new phase of life with confidence and courage. Be not deluded by appearances, nor follow after strange prophets. Let the evolutionary processes work themselves out, and do you fall in with the wave without struggling, and without overmuch striving. The Law is working itself out well—of that be assured. Those who have entered into even a partial understanding and recognition of the One Life underlying, will find that they will be as the chosen people during the changes that are coming to the race. They have attained that which the race is reaching toward in pain and travail. And the force behind the Law will carry them along, for they will be the leaven that is to lighten the great mass of the race in the new dispensation.

Not by deed, or by action, but by Thought, will these people leaven the mass. The Thought is even now at work, and all who read these words are playing a part in the work, although they may know it not. If the race could realize this truth of the One Life underlying, to-day, the Change would occur in a moment, but it will not come in that way. When this understanding gradually dawns upon the race—this new consciousness—then will Things take their proper places, and the Lion and the Lamb lie down together in peace.

We have thought it well to say these things in this the last lesson of this course. They are needed words—they will serve to point out the way to those who are able to read. *"Watch and wait for the Silence that will follow the Storm."*

In this series of lessons, we have endeavored to give you a plain, practical presentation of some of the more important features of "Raja Yoga." But this phase of the subject, as important and interesting as it is, is not the highest phase of the great Yoga teachings. It is merely the preparation of the soil of the mind for what comes afterward. The phase called "Gnani Yoga"—the Yoga of Wisdom—is the highest of all the various phases of Yoga, although each of the lower steps is important in itself. We find ourselves approaching the phase of our work for which we have long wished.

Those who have advised and directed this work have counseled us to deal with the less advanced and simpler phases, in order to prepare the minds of those who might be interested, so that they would be ready for the higher teachings. At times we have felt an impatience for the coming of the day when we would be able to teach the highest that has come to us. And now the time seems to have come. Following this course, we will begin a series of lessons in "GNANI YOGA"—the Yoga of Wisdom—in which we will pass on to our students the highest teachings regarding the Reality and its Manifestations—the One and the Many.

The teachings that "All is Mind" will be explained in such a manner as to be understood by all who have followed us so far. We will be able to impart to you the higher truths about Spiritual Evolution, sometimes called "Reincarnation," as well as Spiritual Cause and Effect, often called "Karma." The highest truths about these important subjects are often obscured by popular misconceptions occasioned by partial teaching. We trust that you—our students—will wish to follow us still higher—higher than we have ventured so far, and we assure you that there is a Truth to be seen and known that is as much higher than the other phases upon which we have touched, as those phases have been higher than the current beliefs of the masses of the race. We trust that the Powers of Knowledge may guide and direct us that we may be able to convey our message so that it may be accepted and understood. We thank our students who have traveled thus far with us, and we assure them that their loving sympathy has ever been a help and an inspiration to us.

Peace be with you.

The Hindu-Yogi Science of Breath

By: William Walker Atkinson

Contents

1 – Salaam

2 – "Breath Is Life"

3 – The Exoteric Theory of Breath

4 – The Esoteric Theory of Breath

5 – The Nervous System

6 – Nostril Breathing vs. Mouth Breathing

7 – The Four Methods of Respiration

8 – How to Acquire the Yogi Complete Breath

9 – Physiological Effect of the Complete Breath

10 – A Few Bits of Yoga Lore

11 – The Seven Yogi Developing Exercises

12 – Seven Minor Yogi Exercises

13 – Vibration and Yogi Rhythmic Breathing

14 – Phenomena of Yogi Psychic Breathing

15 – More Phenomena of Yogi Psychic Breathing

16 – Yogi Spiritual Breathing

CHAPTER 1 - SALAAM

The Western student is apt to be somewhat confused in his ideas regarding the Yogis and their philosophy and practice. Travelers to India have written great tales about the hordes of fakirs, mendicants and mountebanks who infest the great roads of India and the streets of its cities, and who impudently claim the title "Yogi." The Western student is scarcely to be blamed for thinking of the typical Yogi as an emaciated, fanatical, dirty, ignorant Hindu, who either sits in a fixed posture until his body becomes ossified, or else holds his arm up in the air until it becomes stiff and withered and forever after remains in that position, or perhaps clenches his fist and holds it tight until his fingernails grow through the palms of his hands. That these people exist is true, but their claim to the title "Yogi" seems as absurd to the true Yogi as does the claim to the title "Doctor" on the part of the man who pares one's corns seem to the eminent surgeon, or as does the title of "Professor," as assumed by the street corner vendor of worm medicine, seem to the President of Harvard or Yale.

There have been for ages past in India and other Oriental countries men who devoted their time and attention to the development of Man, physically, mentally and spiritually. The experience of generations of earnest seekers has been handed down for centuries from teacher to pupil, and gradually a definite Yogi science was built up. To these investigations and teachings was finally applied the term "Yogi," from the Sanskrit word "Yug," meaning "to join." From the same source comes the English word "yoke," with a similar meaning. Its use in connection with these teachings is difficult to trace, different authorities giving different explanations, but probably the most ingenious is that which holds that it is intended as the Hindu equivalent for the idea conveyed by the English phrase, "getting into harness," or "yoking up," as the Yogi undoubtedly "gets into harness" in his work of controlling the body and mind by the Will.

Yoga is divided into several branches, ranging from that which teaches the control of the body, to that which teaches the attainment of the highest spiritual development. In the work we will not go into the higher phases of the subject, except when the "Science of Breath" touches upon the same. The "Science of Breath" touches Yoga at many points, and although chiefly concerned with the development and control of the physical, has also its psychic side, and even enters the field of spiritual development.

In India there are great schools of Yoga, comprising thousands of the leading minds of that great country. The Yoga philosophy is the rule of life for many people.

The pure Yogi teachings, however, are given only to the few, the masses being satisfied with the crumbs which fall from the tables of the educated classes, the Oriental custom in this respect being opposed to that of the Western world. But Western ideas are beginning to have their effect even in the Orient, and teachings which were once given only to the few are now freely offered to any who are ready to receive them. The East and the West are growing closer together, and both are profiting by the close contact, each influencing the other.

The Hindu Yogis have always paid great attention to the Science of Breath, for reasons which will be apparent to the student who reads this book. Many Western writers have touched upon this phase of the Yogi teachings, but we believe that it has been reserved for the writer of this work to give to the Western student, in concise form and simple language, the underlying principles of the Yogi Science of Breath, together with many of the favorite Yogi breathing exercises and methods. We have given the Western idea as well as the Oriental, showing how one dovetails into the other. We have used the ordinary English terms, almost entirely, avoiding the Sanskrit terms, so confusing to the average Western reader.

The first part of the book is devoted to the physical phase of the Science of Breath; then the psychic and mental sides are considered, and finally the spiritual side is touched upon.

We may be pardoned if we express ourselves as pleased with our success in condensing so much Yogi lore into so few pages, and by the use of words and terms which may be understood by anyone. Our only fear is that its very simplicity may cause some to pass it by as unworthy of attention, while they pass on their way searching for something "deep," mysterious and non-understandable. However, the Western mind is eminently practical, and we know that it is only a question of a short time before it will recognize the practicability of this work.

We greet our students, with our most profound salaam, and bid them be seated for their first lessons in the Yogi Science of Breath.

CHAPTER 2 - "BREATH IS LIFE"

Life is absolutely dependent upon the act of breathing. "Breath is Life."

Differ as they may upon details of theory and terminology, the Oriental and the Occidental agree upon these fundamental principles.

To breathe is to live, and without breath there is no life. Not only are the higher animals dependent upon breath for life and health, but even the lower forms of animal life must breathe to live, and plant life is likewise dependent upon the air for continued existence.

The infant draws in a long, deep breath, retains it for a moment to extract from it its life-giving properties, and then exhales it in a long wail, and lo! its life upon earth has begun. The old man gives a faint gasp, ceases to breathe, and life is over. From the first faint breath of the infant to the last gasp of the dying man, it is one long story of continued breathing. Life is but a series of breaths.

Breathing may be considered the most important of all of the functions of the body, for, indeed, all the other functions depend upon it. Man may exist some time without eating; a shorter time without drinking; but without breathing his existence may be measured by a few minutes.

And not only is Man dependent upon Breath for life, but he is largely dependent upon correct habits of breathing for continued vitality and freedom from disease. An intelligent control of our breathing power will lengthen our days upon earth by giving us increased vitality and powers of resistance, and, on the other hand, unintelligent and careless breathing will tend to shorten our days, by decreasing our vitality and laying us open to disease.

Man in his normal state had no need of instruction in breathing. Like the lower animal and the child, he breathed naturally and properly, as nature intended him to do, but civilization has changed him in this and other respects. He has contracted improper methods and attitudes of walking, standing and sitting, which have robbed him of his birthright of natural and correct breathing. He has paid a high price for civilization. The savage, to-day, breathes naturally, unless he has been contaminated by the habits of civilized man.

The percentage of civilized men who breathe correctly is quite small, and the result is shown in contracted chests and stooping shoulders, and the terrible increase in diseases of the respiratory organs, including that dread monster, Consumption, "the white scourge." Eminent authorities have stated that one generation of correct breathers would regenerate the race, and disease would be so rare as to be looked upon as a curiosity. Whether looked at from the standpoint of the Oriental or Occidental, the connection between correct breathing and health is readily seen and explained.

The Occidental teachings show that the physical health depends very materially upon correct breathing. The Oriental teachers not only admit that their Occidental brothers are right, but say that in addition to the physical benefit derived from correct habits of breathing, Man's mental power, happiness, self-control, clear-sightedness, morals, and even his spiritual growth may be increased by an understanding of the "Science of Breath." Whole schools of Oriental Philosophy have been founded upon this science, and this knowledge when grasped by the Western races, and by them put to the practical use which is their strong point, will work wonders among them. The theory of the East, wedded to the practice of the West, will produce worthy offspring.

This work will take up the Yogi "Science of Breath," which includes not only all that is known to the Western physiologist and hygienist, but the occult side of the subject as well. It not only points out the way to physical health along the lines of what Western scientists have termed "deep breathing," etc., but also goes into the less known phases of the subject, and shows how the Hindu Yogi controls his body, increasing his mental capacity, and develops the spiritual side of his nature by the "Science of Breath."

The Yogi practices exercises by which he attains control of his body, and is enabled to send to any organ or part an increased flow of vital force or "prana," thereby strengthening and invigorating the part or organ. He knows all that his Western scientific brother knows about the physiological effect of correct breathing, but he also knows that the air contains more than oxygen and hydrogen and nitrogen, and that something more is accomplished than the mere oxygenating of the blood. He knows something about "prana," of which his Western brother is ignorant, and he is fully aware of the nature and manner of handling that great principle of energy, and is fully informed as to its effect upon the human body and mind. He knows that by rhythmical breathing one may bring himself into harmonious vibration with nature, and aid in the unfoldment of his latent powers. He knows that by controlled breathing he may not only cure disease in himself and others, but also practically do away with fear and worry and the baser emotions.

To teach these things is the object of this work. We will give in a few chapters concise explanations and instructions, which might be extended into volumes. We hope to awaken the minds of the Western world to the value of the Yogi "Science of Breath."

CHAPTER 3 - THE EXOTERIC THEORY OF BREATH

In this chapter we will give you briefly the theories of the Western scientific world regarding the functions of the respiratory organs, and the part in the human economy played by the breath. In subsequent chapters we will give the additional theories and ascertained facts of the Oriental school of thought and research. The Oriental accepts the theories and facts of his Western brothers (which have been known to him for centuries) and adds thereto much that the latter do not now accept, but which they will in due time "discover" and which, after renaming, they will present to the world as a great truth.

Before taking up the Western idea, it will perhaps be better to give a hasty general idea of the Organs of Respiration.

The Organs of Respiration consist of the lungs and the air passages leading to them. The lungs are two in number, and occupy the pleural chamber of the thorax, one on each side of the median line, being separated from each other by the heart, the greater blood vessels and the larger air tubes. Each lung is free in all directions, except at the root, which consists chiefly of the bronchi, arteries and veins connecting the lungs with the trachea and heart. The lungs are spongy and porous, and their tissues are very elastic. They are covered with a delicately constructed but strong sac, known as the pleural sac, one wall of which closely adheres to the lung, and the other to the inner wall of the chest, and which secretes a fluid which allows the inner surfaces of the walls to glide easily upon each other in the act of breathing.

The Air Passages consist of the interior of the nose, pharynx, larynx, windpipe or trachea, and the bronchial tubes. When we breathe, we draw in the air through the nose, in which it is warmed by contact with the mucous membrane, which is richly supplied with blood, and after it has passed through the pharynx and larynx it passes into the trachea or windpipe, which subdivides into numerous tubes called the bronchial tubes (bronchia), which in turn subdivide into and terminate in minute subdivisions in all the small air spaces in the lungs, of which the lungs contain millions. A writer has stated that if the air cells of the lungs were spread out over an unbroken surface, they would cover an area of fourteen thousand square feet.

The air is drawn into the lungs by the action of the diaphragm, a great, strong, flat, sheet-like muscle, stretched across the chest, separating the chest-box from the abdomen. The diaphragm's action is almost as automatic as that of the heart, although it may be transformed into a semi-voluntary muscle by an effort of the will. When it expands, it increases the size of the chest and lungs, and the air rushes into the vacuum thus created. When it relaxes the chest and lungs contract and the air is expelled from the lungs.

Now, before considering what happens to the air in the lungs, let us look a little into the matter of the circulation of the blood. The blood, as you know, is driven by the heart, through the arteries, into the capillaries, thus reaching every part of the body, which it vitalizes, nourishes and strengthens. It then returns by means of the capillaries by another route, the veins, to the heart, from whence it is drawn to the lungs.

The blood starts on its arterial journey, bright red and rich, laden with life-giving qualities and properties. It returns by the venous route, poor, blue and dull, being laden down with the waste matter of the system. It goes out like a fresh stream from the mountains; it returns as a stream of sewer water. This foul stream goes to the right auricle of the heart. When this auricle becomes filled, it contracts and forces the stream of blood through an opening in the right ventricle of the heart, which in turn sends it on to the lungs, where it is distributed by millions of hair-like blood vessels to the air cells of the lungs, of which we have spoken. Now, let us take up the story of the lungs at this point.

The foul stream of blood is now distributed among the millions of tiny air cells in the lungs. A breath of air is inhaled and the oxygen of the air comes in contact with the impure blood through the thin walls of the hair-like blood vessels of the lungs, which walls are thick enough to hold the blood, but thin enough to admit the oxygen to penetrate them. When the oxygen comes in contact with the blood, a form of combustion takes place, and the blood takes up oxygen and releases carbonic acid gas generated from the waste products and poisonous matter which has been gathered up by the blood from all parts of the system.

The blood thus purified and oxygenated is carried back to the heart, again rich, red and bright, and laden with life-giving properties and qualities. Upon reaching the left auricle of the heart, it is forced into the left ventricle, from whence it is again forced out through the arteries on its mission of life to all parts of the system. It is estimated that in a single day of twenty-four hours, 35,000 pints of blood traverse the capillaries of the lungs, the blood corpuscles passing in single file and being exposed to the oxygen of the air on both of their surfaces. When one considers the minute details of the process alluded to, he is lost in wonder and admiration at Nature's infinite care and intelligence.

It will be seen that unless fresh air in sufficient quantities reaches the lungs, the foul stream of venous blood cannot be purified, and consequently not only is the body thus robbed of nourishment, but the waste products which should have been destroyed are returned to the circulation and poison the system, and death ensues. Impure air acts in the same way, only in a lessened degree. It will also be seen that if one does not breathe in a sufficient quantity of air, the work of the blood cannot go on properly, and the result is that the body is insufficiently nourished and disease ensues, or a state of imperfect health is experienced. The blood of one who breathes improperly is, of course, of a bluish, dark color, lacking the rich redness of pure arterial blood. This often shows itself in a poor complexion. Proper breathing, and a consequent good circulation, results in a clear, bright complexion.

A little reflection will show the vital importance of correct breathing. If the blood is not fully purified by the regenerative process of the lungs, it returns to the arteries in an abnormal state, insufficiently purified and imperfectly cleansed of the impurities which it took up on its return journey. These impurities if returned to the system will certainly manifest in some form of disease, either in a form of blood disease or some disease resulting from impaired functioning of some insufficiently nourished organ or tissue.

The blood, when properly exposed to the air in the lungs, not only has its impurities consumed, and parts with its noxious carbonic acid gas, but it also takes up and absorbs a certain quantity of oxygen which it carries to all parts of the body, where it is needed in order that Nature may perform her processes properly. When the oxygen comes in contact with the blood, it unites with the hemoglobin of the blood and is carried to every cell, tissue, muscle and organ, which it invigorates and strengthens, replacing the worn-out cells and tissue by new materials which Nature converts to her use. Arterial blood, properly exposed to the air, contains about 25 per cent of free oxygen.

Not only is every part vitalized by the oxygen, but the act of digestion depends materially upon a certain amount of oxygenation of the food, and this can be accomplished only by the oxygen in the blood coming in contact with the food and producing a certain form of combustion. It is therefore necessary that a proper supply of oxygen be taken through the lungs. This accounts for the fact that weak lungs and poor digestion are so often found together. To grasp the full significance of this statement, one must remember that the entire body receives nourishment from the food assimilated, and that imperfect assimilation always means an imperfectly nourished body. Even the lungs themselves depend upon the same source for nourishment, and if through imperfect breathing the assimilation becomes imperfect, and the lungs in turn become weakened, they are rendered still less able to perform their work properly, and so in turn the body becomes further weakened.

Every particle of food and drink must be oxygenated before it can yield us the proper nourishment, and before the waste products of the system can be reduced to the proper condition to be eliminated from the system. Lack of sufficient oxygen means Imperfect nutrition, Imperfect elimination and imperfect health. Verily, "breath is life."

The combustion arising from the change in the waste products generates heat and equalizes the temperature of the body. Good breathers are not apt to "take cold," and they generally have plenty of good warm blood which enables them to resist the changes in the outer temperature.

In addition to the above-mentioned important processes the act of breathing gives exercise to the internal organs and muscles, which feature is generally overlooked by the Western writers on the subject, but which the Yogis fully appreciate.

In imperfect or shallow breathing, only a portion of the lung cells are brought into play, and a great portion of the lung capacity is lost, the system suffering in proportion to the amount of under-oxygenation. The lower animals, in their native state, breathe naturally, and primitive man undoubtedly did the same. The abnormal manner of living adopted by civilized man—the shadow that follows upon civilization—has robbed us of our natural habit of breathing, and the race has greatly suffered thereby. Man's only physical salvation is to "get back to Nature."

CHAPTER 4 - THE ESOTERIC THEORY OF BREATH

The Science of Breath, like many other teachings, has its esoteric or inner phase, as well as its exoteric or external. The physiological phase may be termed the outer or exoteric side of the subject, and the phase which we will now consider may be termed its esoteric or inner side. Occultists, in all ages and lands, have always taught, usually secretly to a few followers, that there was to be found in the air a substance or principle from which all activity, vitality and life was derived. They differed in their terms and names for this force, as well as in the details of the theory, but the main principle is to be found in all occult teachings and philosophies, and has for centuries formed a portion of the teachings of the Oriental Yogis.

In order to avoid misconceptions arising from the various theories regarding this great principle, which theories are usually attached to some name given the principle, we, in this work, will speak of the principle as "Prana," this word being the Sanskrit term meaning "Absolute Energy." Many occult authorities teach that the principle which the Hindus term "Prana" is the universal principle of energy or force, and that all energy or force is derived from that principle, or, rather, is a particular form of manifestation of that principle. These theories do not concern us in the consideration of the subject matter of this work, and we will therefore confine ourselves to an understanding of prana as the principle of energy exhibited in all living things, which distinguishes them from a lifeless thing. We may consider it as the active principle of life—Vital Force, if you please.

It is found in all forms of life, from the amoeba to man—from the most elementary form of plant life to the highest form of animal life. Prana is all pervading. It is found in all things having life, and as the occult philosophy teaches that life is in all things—in every atom—the apparent lifelessness of some things being only a lesser degree of manifestation, we may understand their teachings that prana is everywhere, in everything. Prana must not be confounded with the Ego— that bit of Divine Spirit in every soul, around which clusters matter and energy.

Prana is merely a form of energy used by the Ego in its material manifestation. When the Ego leaves the body, the prana, being no longer under its control, responds only to the orders of the individual atoms, or groups of atoms, forming the body, and as the body disintegrates and is resolved to its original elements, each atom takes with it sufficient prana to enable it to form new combinations, the unused prana returning to the great universal storehouse from which it came. With the Ego in control, cohesion exists and the atoms are held together by the Will of the Ego.

Prana is the name by which we designate a universal principle, which principle is the essence of all motion, force or energy, whether manifested in gravitation, electricity, the revolution of the planets, and all forms of life, from the highest to the lowest. It may be called the soul of Force and Energy in all their forms, and that principle which, operating in a certain way, causes that form of activity which accompanies Life.

This great principle is in all forms of matter, and yet it is not matter. It is in the air, but it is not the air nor one of its chemical constituents. Animal and plant life breathe it in with the air, and yet if the air didn't contained it, they would die even though they might be filled with air. It is taken up by the system along with the oxygen, and yet is not the oxygen. The Hebrew writer of the book of Genesis knew the difference between the atmospheric air and the mysterious and potent principle contained within it. He speaks of neshemet ruach chayim, which, translated, means "the breath of the spirit of life." In the Hebrew neshemet means the ordinary breath of atmospheric air, and chayim means life or lives, while the word ruach means the "spirit of life," which occultists claim is the same principle which we speak of as Prana.

Prana is in the atmospheric air, but it is also elsewhere, and it penetrates where the air cannot reach. The oxygen in the air plays an important part in sustaining animal life, and the carbon plays a similar part with plant life, but Prana has its own distinct part to play in the manifestation of life, aside from the physiological functions.

We are constantly inhaling the air charged with prana, and are as constantly extracting the latter from the air and appropriating it to our uses. Prana is found in its freest state in the atmospheric air, which when fresh is fairly charged with it, and we draw it to us more easily from the air than from any other source. In ordinary breathing we absorb and extract a normal supply of prana, but by controlled and regulated breathing (generally known as Yogi breathing) we are enabled to extract a greater supply, which is stored away in the brain and nerve centers, to be used when necessary. We may store away prana, just as the storage battery stores away electricity. The many powers attributed to advanced occultists is due largely to their knowledge of this fact and their intelligent use of this stored-up energy.

The Yogis know that by certain forms of breathing they establish certain relations with the supply of prana and may draw on the same for what they require. Not only do they strengthen all parts of their body in this way, but the brain itself may receive increased energy from the same source, and latent faculties be developed and psychic powers attained. One who has mastered the science of storing away prana, either consciously or unconsciously, often radiates vitality and strength which is felt by those coming in contact with him, and such a person may impart this strength to others, and give them increased vitality and health. What is called "magnetic healing" is performed in this way, although many practitioners are not aware of the source of their power.

Western scientists have been dimly aware of this great principle with which the air is charged, but finding that they could find no chemical trace of it, or make it register an any of their instruments, they have generally treated the Oriental theory with disdain. They could not explain this principle, and so denied it. They seem, however, to recognize that the air in certain places possesses a greater amount of "something" and sick people are directed by their physicians to seek such places in hopes of regaining, lost health.

The oxygen in the air is appropriated by the blood and is made use of by the circulatory system. The prana in the air is appropriated by the nervous system, and is used in its work. And as the oxygenated blood is carried to all parts of the system, building up and replenishing, so is the prana carried to all parts of the nervous system, adding strength and vitality. If we think of prana as being the active principle of what we call "vitality," we will be able to form a much clearer idea of what an important part it plays in our lives. Just as is the oxygen in the blood used up by the wants of the system, so the supply of prana taken up by the nervous system is exhausted by our thinking, willing, acting, etc., and in consequence constant replenishing is necessary.

Every thought, every act, every effort of the will, every motion of a muscle, uses up a certain amount of what we call nerve force, which is really a form of prana. To move a muscle the brain sends out an impulse over the nerves, and the muscle contracts, and so much prana is expended. When it is remembered that the greater portion of prana acquired by man comes to him from the air inhaled, the importance of proper breathing is readily understood.

CHAPTER 5 - THE NERVOUS SYSTEM

It will be noticed that the Western scientific theories regarding the breath confine themselves to the effects of the absorption of oxygen, and its use through the circulatory system, while the Yogi theory also takes into consideration the absorption of Prana, and its manifestation through the channels of the Nervous System. Before proceeding further, it may be as well to take a hasty glance at the Nervous System.

The Nervous System of man is divided into two great systems, viz., the Cerebro-Spinal System and the Sympathetic System. The Cerebro-Spinal System consists of all that part of the Nervous System contained within the cranial cavity and the spinal canal, viz., the brain and the spinal cord, together with the nerves which branch off from the same. This system presides over the functions of animal life known as volition, sensation, etc. The Sympathetic System includes all that part of the Nervous System located principally in the thoracic, abdominal and pelvic cavities, and which is distributed to the internal organs. It has control over the involuntary processes, such as growth, nutrition, etc.

The Cerebro-Spinal System attends to all the seeing, hearing, tasting, smelling, feeling, etc. It sets things in motion; it is used by the Ego to think—to manifest consciousness. It is the instrument with which the Ego communicates with the outside world. This system may be likened to a telephone system, with the brain as the central office, and the spinal column and nerves as cable and wires respectively.

The brain is a great mass of nerve tissue, and consists of three parts, viz., the Cerebrum or brain proper, which occupies the upper, front, middle and back portion of the skull; the Cerebellum, or "little brain," which fills the lower and back portion of the skull; and the Medulla Oblongata, which Is the broadened commencement of the spinal cord, lying before and in front of the Cerebellum.

The Cerebrum is the organ of that part of the mind which manifests itself in intellectual action. The Cerebellum regulates the movements of the voluntary muscles. The Medulla Oblongata is the upper enlarged end of the spinal cord, and from it and the Cerebrum branch forth the Cranial Nerves which reach to various parts of the head, to the organs of special sense, and to some of the thoracic and abdominal organs, and to the organs of respiration.

The Spinal Cord, or spinal marrow, fills the spinal canal in the vertebral column, or "backbone." It is a long mass of nerve tissue, branching off at the several vertebrae to nerves communicating with all parts of the body. The Spinal Cord is like a large telephone cable, and the emerging nerves are like the private wires connecting therewith.

The Sympathetic Nervous System consists of a double chain of Ganglia on the side of the Spinal column, and scattered ganglia in the head, neck, chest and abdomen. (A ganglion is a mass of nervous matter including nerve cells.) These ganglia are connected with each other by filaments, and are also connected with the Cerebro-Spinal System by motor and sensory nerves. From these ganglia numerous fibers branch out to the organs of the body, blood vessels, etc. At various points, the nerves meet together and form what are known as plexuses. The Sympathetic System practically controls the involuntary processes, such as circulation, respiration and digestion.

The power or force transmitted from the brain to all parts of the body by means of the nerves, is known to Western science as "nerve force," although the Yogi knows it to be a manifestation of Prana. In character and rapidity, it resembles the electric current. It will be seen that without this "nerve force" the heart cannot beat; the blood cannot circulate; the lungs cannot breathe; the various organs cannot function; in fact, the machinery of the body comes to a stop without it. Nay more, even the brain cannot think without Prana be present. When these facts are considered, the importance of the absorption of Prana must be evident to all, and the Science of Breath assumes an importance even greater than that accorded it by Western science.

The Yogi teachings go further than does Western science, in one important feature of the Nervous System. We allude to what Western science terms the "Solar Plexus," and which it considers as merely one of a series of certain matted nets of sympathetic nerves with their ganglia found in various parts of the body. Yogi science teaches that this Solar Plexus is really a most important part of the Nervous System, and that it is a form of brain, playing one of the principal parts in the human economy. Western science seems to be moving gradually towards a recognition of this fact which has been known to the Yogis of the East for centuries, and some recent Western writers have termed the Solar Plexus the "Abdominal Brain."

The Solar Plexus is situated in the Epigastric region, just back of the "pit of the stomach" on either side of the spinal column. It is composed of white and gray brain matter, similar to that composing the other brains of man. It has control of the main internal organs of man, and plays a much more important part than is generally recognized. We will not go into the Yogi theory regarding the Solar Plexus, further than to say that they know it as the great central store-house of Prana. Men have been known to be instantly killed by a severe blow over the Solar Plexus, and prize fighters recognize its vulnerability and frequently temporarily paralyze their opponents by a blow over this region.

The name "Solar" is well bestowed on this "brain," as it radiates strength and energy to all parts of the body, even the upper brains depending largely upon it as a storehouse of Prana. Sooner or later Western science will fully recognize the real function of the Solar Plexus, and will accord to it a far more important place then it now occupies in their text-books and teachings.

CHAPTER 6 - NOSTRIL-BREATHING VS. MOUTH-BREATHING

One of the first lessons in the Yogi Science of Breath, is to learn how to breathe through the nostrils, and to overcome the common practice of mouth-breathing.

The breathing mechanism of Man is so constructed that he may breathe either through the mouth or nasal tubes, but it is a matter of vital importance to him which method he follows, as one brings health and strength and the other disease and weakness.

It should not be necessary to state to the student that the proper method of breathing is to take the breath through the nostrils, but alas! the ignorance among civilized people regarding this simple matter is astounding. We find people in all walks of life habitually breathing through their mouths, and allowing their children to follow their horrible and disgusting example.

Many of the diseases to which civilized man is subject are undoubtedly caused by this common habit of mouth-breathing. Children permitted to breathe in this way grow up with impaired vitality and weakened constitutions, and in manhood and womanhood break down and become chronic invalids. The mother of the savage race does better, being evidently guided by her intuition. She seems to instinctively recognize that the nostrils are the proper channels for the movement of air to the lungs, and she trains her infant to close its little lips and breathe through the nose. She tips its head forward when it is asleep, which attitude closes the lips and makes nostril-breathing imperative. If our civilized mothers were to adopt the same plan, it would work a great good for the race.

Many contagious diseases are contracted by the disgusting habit of mouth-breathing, and many cases of cold and catarrhal affections are also attributable to the same cause. Many persons who, for the sake of appearances, keep their mouth closed during the day, persist in mouth-breathing at night and often contract disease in this way.

Carefully conducted scientific experiments have shown that soldiers and sailors who sleep with their mouths open are much more liable to contract contagious diseases than those who breathe properly through the nostrils. An instance is related in which small-pox became epidemic on a man-of-war in foreign parts, and every death which resulted was that of some sailor or marine who was a mouth-breather, not a single nostril-breather succumbing.

The organs of respiration have their only protective apparatus, filter, or dust-catcher, in the nostrils. When the breath is taken through the mouth, there is nothing from mouth to lungs to strain the air, or to catch the dust and other foreign matter in the air. From mouth to lungs the dirt or impure substance has a clear track, and the entire respiratory system is unprotected. And, moreover, such incorrect breathing admits cold air to the organs, thereby injuring them. Inflammation of the respiratory organs often results from the inhalation of cold air through the mouth. The man who breathes through the mouth at night, always awakens with a parched feeling in the mouth and a dryness in the throat. He is violating one of nature's laws, and is sowing the seeds of disease.

Once more, remember that the mouth affords no protection to the respiratory organs, and cold air, dust and impurities and germs readily enter by that door. On the other hand, the nostrils and nasal passages show evidence of the careful design of nature in this respect. The nostrils are two narrow, tortuous channels, containing numerous bristly hairs which serve the purpose of a filter or sieve to strain the air of its impurities, etc., which are expelled when the breath is exhaled. Not only do the nostrils serve this important purpose, but they also perform an important function in warming the air inhaled. The long narrow winding nostrils are filled with warm mucous membrane, which coming in contact with the inhaled air Warms it so that it can do no damage to the delicate organs of the throat, or to the lungs.

No animal, excepting man, sleeps with the mouth open or breathes through the mouth, and in fact it is believed that it is only civilized man who so perverts nature's functions, as the savage and barbarian races almost invariably breathe correctly. It is probable that this unnatural habit among civilized men has been acquired through unnatural methods of living, enervating luxuries and excessive warmth.

The refining, filtering and straining apparatus of the nostrils renders the air fit to reach the delicate organs of the throat and the lungs, and the air is not fit to so reach these organs until it has passed through nature's refining process. The impurities which are stopped and retained by the sieves and mucous membrane of the nostrils, are thrown out again by the expelled breath, in exhalation, and in case they have accumulated too rapidly or have managed to escape through the sieves and have penetrated forbidden regions, nature protects us by producing a sneeze which violently ejects the intruder.

The air, when it enters the lungs is as different from the outside air, as is distilled water different from the water of the cistern. The intricate purifying organization of the nostrils, arresting and holding the impure particles in the air, is as important as is the action of the mouth in stopping cherry-stones and fish-bones and preventing them from being carried on to the stomach. Man should no more breathe through his mouth than he would attempt to take food through his nose.

Another feature of mouth-breathing is that the nasal passages, being thus comparatively unused, consequently fail to keep themselves clean and clear, and become clogged up and unclean, and are apt to contract local diseases. Like abandoned roads that soon become filled with weeds and rubbish, unused nostrils become filled with impurities and foul matter.

One who habitually breathes through the nostrils is not likely to be troubled with clogged or stuffy nostrils, but for the benefit of those who have been more or less addicted to the unnatural mouth-breathing, and who wish to acquire the natural and rational method, it may perhaps be well to add a few words regarding the way to keep their nostrils clean and free from impurities.

A favorite Oriental method is to snuff a little water up the nostrils allowing it to run down the passage into the throat, from thence it may be ejected through the mouth. Some Hindu yogis immerse the face in a bowl of water, and by a sort of suction draw in quite a quantity of water, but this latter method requires considerable practice, and the first mentioned method is equally efficacious, and much more easily performed.

Another good plan is to open the window and breathe freely, closing one nostril with the finger or thumb, sniffing up the air through the open nostril. Then repeat the process on the other nostril. Repeat several times, changing nostrils. This method will usually clear the nostrils of obstructions.

In case the trouble is caused by catarrh it is well to apply a little Vaseline or camphor ice or similar preparation. Or sniff up a little witch-hazel extract once in a while, and you will notice a marked improvement. A little care and attention will result in the nostrils becoming clean and remaining so.

We have given considerable space to this subject of nostril-breathing, not only because of its great importance in its reference to health, but because nostril-breathing is a prerequisite to the practice of the breathing exercises to be given later in this book, and because nostril-breathing is one of the basic principles underlying the Yogi Science of Breath.

We urge upon the student the necessity of acquiring this method of breathing if he has it not, and caution him against dismissing this phase of the subject as unimportant.

CHAPTER 7 - FOUR METHODS OF RESPIRATION

In the consideration of the question of respiration, we must begin by considering the mechanical arrangements whereby the respiratory movements are affected. The mechanics of respiration manifest through (1) the elastic movements of the lungs, and (2) the activities of the sides and bottom of the thoracic cavity in which the lungs are contained. The thorax is that portion of the trunk between the neck and the abdomen, the cavity of which (known as the thoracic cavity) is occupied mainly by the lungs and heart. It is bounded by the spinal column, the ribs with their cartilages, the breastbone, and below by the diaphragm. It is generally spoken of as "the chest." It has been compared to a completely shut, conical box, the small end of which Is turned upward, the back of the box being formed by the spinal column, the front by the breastbone and the sides by the ribs.

The ribs are twenty-four in number, twelve on each side, and emerge from each side of the spinal column. The upper seven pair are known as "true ribs," being fastened to the breastbone direct, while the lower five pairs are called (false ribs) or "floating ribs," because they are not so fastened, the upper two of them being fastened by cartilage to the other ribs, the remainder having no cartilages, their forward ends being free.

The ribs are moved in respiration by two superficial muscular layers, known as the intercostal muscles. The diaphragm, the muscular partition before alluded to, separates the chest box from the abdominal cavity.

In the act of inhalation, the muscles expand the lungs so that a vacuum is created and the air rushes in in accordance with the well-known law of physics. Everything depends upon the muscles concerned in the process of respiration, which we may as, for convenience, term the "respiratory muscles." Without the aid of these muscles the lungs cannot expand, and upon the proper use and control of these muscles the Science of Breath largely depends. The proper control of these muscles will result in the ability to attain the maximum degree of lung expansion, and the greatest amount of the life-giving properties of the air into the system.

The Yogis classify Respiration into four general methods, viz:

(1) High Breathing.

(2) Mid Breathing.

(3) Low Breathing.

(4) Yogi Complete Breathing.

We will give a general idea of the first three methods, and a more extended treatment of the fourth method, upon which the Yogi Science of Breath is largely based.

(1) HIGH BREATHING

This form of breathing is known to the Western world as Clavicular Breathing, or Collarbone Breathing. One breathing in this way elevates the ribs and raises the collarbone and shoulders, at the same time drawing in the abdomen and pushing its contents up against the diaphragm, which in turn is raised.

The upper part of the chest and lungs, which is the smallest, is used, and consequently but a minimum amount of air enters the lungs. In addition to this, the diaphragm being raised, there can be no expansion in that direction. A study of the anatomy of the chest will convince any student that in this way a maximum amount of effort is used to obtain a minimum amount of benefit.

High Breathing is probably the worst form of breathing known to man and requires the greatest expenditure of energy with the smallest amount of benefit. It is an energy-wasting, poor-returns plan. It is quite common among the Western races, many women being addicted to It, and even singers, clergymen, lawyers and others, who should know better, using it ignorantly.

Many diseases of the vocal organs and organs of respiration may be directly traced to this barbarous method of breathing, and the straining of delicate organs caused by this method, often results in the harsh, disagreeable voices heard on all sides. Many persons who breathe in this way become addicted to the disgusting practice of "mouth-breathing" described in a preceding chapter.

If the student has any doubts about what has been said regarding this form of breathing, let him try the experiment of expelling all the air from his lungs, then standing erect, with hands at sides, let him raise the shoulders and collar-bone and inhale. He will find that the amount of air inhaled far below normal. Then let him inhale a full breath, after dropping the shoulders and collar-bone, and he will receive an object lesson in breathing which he will be apt to remember much longer than he would any words, printed or spoken.

(2) MID BREATHING

This method of respiration is known to Western students as Rib Breathing, or Inter-Costal Breathing, and while less objectionable than High Breathing, is far inferior to either Low Breathing or to the Yogi Complete Breath. In Mid Breathing the diaphragm is pushed upward, and the abdomen drawn in. The ribs are raised somewhat, and the chest is partially expanded. It is quite common among men who have made no study of the subject. As there are two better methods known, we give it only passing notice, and that principally to call your attention to its short-comings.

(3) LOW BREATHING

This form of respiration is far better than either of the two preceding forms: and of recent years many Western writers have extolled its merits, and have exploited it under the names of "Abdominal Breathing," "Deep Breathing," "Diaphragmatic Breathing," etc., etc., and much good has been accomplished by the attention of the public having been directed to the subject, and many having been Induced to substitute it for the interior and injurious methods above alluded to. Many "systems" of breathing have been built around Low Breathing, and students have paid high prices to learn the new (?) systems. But, as we have said, much good has resulted, and after all the students who paid high prices to learn revamped old systems undoubtedly got their money's worth if they were Induced to discard the old methods of High Breathing and Low Breathing.

Although many Western authorities write and speak of this method as the best-known form of breathing, the Yogis know it to be but a part of a system which they have used for centuries and which they know as "The Complete Breath." It must be admitted, however, that one must be acquainted with the principles of Low Breathing before he can grasp the idea of Complete Breathing.

Let us again consider the diaphragm. What is it? We have seen that it is the great partition muscle, which separates the chest and its contents from the abdomen and its contents. When at rest it presents a concave surface to the abdomen. That is, the diaphragm as viewed from the abdomen would seem like the sky as viewed from the earth—the interior of an arched surface. Consequently, the side of the diaphragm toward the chest organs is like a protruding rounded surface—like a hill. When the diaphragm is brought into use the hill formation is lowered and the diaphragm presses upon the abdominal organs and forces out the abdomen.

In Low Breathing, the lungs are given freer play than in the methods already mentioned, and consequently more air is inhaled. This fact has led the majority of Western writers to speak and write of Low Breathing (which they call Abdominal Breathing) as the highest and best method known to science. But the Oriental Yogi has long known of a better method, and some few Western writers have also recognized this fact. The trouble with all methods of breathing, other than "Yogi

Complete Breathing" is that in none of these methods do the lungs become filled with air—at the best only a portion of the lung space is filled, even in Low Breathing. High Breathing fills only the upper portion of the lungs. Mid Breathing fills only the middle and a portion of the upper parts. Low Breathing fills only the lower and middle parts. It is evident that any method that fills the entire lung space must be far preferable to those filling only certain parts Any method which will fill the entire lung space must be the greatest value to Man in the way of allowing him to absorb the greatest quantity of oxygen and to store away the greatest amount of prana. The Complete Breath is known to the Yogis to be the best method of respiration known to science.

THE YOGI COMPLETE BREATH

Yogi Complete Breathing includes all the good points of High Breathing, Mid Breathing and Low Breathing, with the objectionable features of each eliminated. It brings into play the entire respiratory apparatus, every part of the lungs, every air-cell, every respiratory muscle. The entire respiratory organism responds to this method of breathing, and the maximum amount of benefit is derived from the minimum expenditure of energy. The chest cavity is increased to its normal limits in all directions and every part of the machinery performs its natural work and functions.

One of the most important features of this method of breathing is the fact that the respiratory muscles are fully called into play, whereas in the other forms of breathing only a portion of these muscles are so used. In Complete Breathing, among other muscles, those controlling the ribs are actively used, which increases the space in which the lungs may expand, and also gives the proper support to the organs when needed, Nature availing herself of the perfection of the principle of leverage in this process. Certain muscles hold the lower ribs firmly in position, while other muscles bend them outward.

Then again, in this method, the diaphragm is under perfect control and is able to perform its functions properly, and in such manner as to yield the maximum degree of service.

In the rib-action, above alluded to, the lower ribs are controlled by the diaphragm which draws them slightly downward, while other muscles hold them in place and the intercostal muscles force them outward, which combined action increases the mid-chest cavity to its maximum. In addition to this muscular action, the upper ribs are also lifted and forced outward by the intercostal muscles, which increases the capacity of the upper chest to its fullest extent.

If you have studied the special features of the four given methods of breathing, you will at once see that the Complete Breath comprises all the advantageous features of the three other methods, plus the reciprocal advantages accruing from the combined action of the high-chest, mid-chest, and diaphragmatic regions, and the normal rhythm thus obtained.

In our next chapter, we will take up the Complete Breath in practice, and will give full directions for the acquirement of this superior method of breathing, with exercises, etc.

CHAPTER 8 - HOW TO ACQUIRE THE YOGI COMPLETE BREATH

The Yogi Complete Breath is the fundamental breath of the entire Yogi Science of Breath, and the student must fully acquaint himself with it, and master it perfectly before he can hope to obtain results from the other forms of breath-mentioned and given in this book. He should not be content with half-learning it, but should go to work in earnest until it becomes his natural method of breathing. This will require work, time and patience, but without these things nothing is ever accomplished. There is no royal road to the Science of Breath, and the student must be prepared to practice and study in earnest if he expects to receive results.

The results obtained by a complete mastery of the Science of Breath are great, and no one who has attained them would willingly go back to the old methods, and he will tell his friends that he considers himself amply repaid for all his work. We say these things now, that you may fully understand the necessity and importance of mastering this fundamental method of Yogi Breathing, instead of passing it by and trying some of the attractive looking variations given later on in this book. Again, we say to you: Start right, and right results will follow; but neglect your foundations and your entire building will topple over sooner or later.

Perhaps the better way to teach you how to develop the Yogi Complete Breath, would be to give you simple directions regarding the breath itself, and then follow up the same with general remarks concerning it, and then later on giving exercises for developing the chest, muscles and lungs which have been allowed to remain in an undeveloped condition by imperfect methods of breathing. Right here we wish to say that this Complete Breath is not a forced or abnormal thing, but on the contrary is a going back to first principles—a return to Nature.

The healthy adult savage and the healthy infant of civilization both breathe in this manner, but civilized man has adopted unnatural methods of living, clothing, etc., and has lost his birthright. And we wish to remind the reader that the Complete Breath does not necessarily call for the complete filling of the lungs at every inhalation.

One may inhale the average amount of air, using the Complete Breathing Method and distributing the air inhaled, be the quantity large or small, to all parts of the lungs. But one should inhale a series of full Complete Breaths several times a day, whenever opportunity offers, in order to keep the system in good order and condition.

The following simple exercise will give you a clear idea of what the Complete Breath is:

(1) Stand or sit erect. Breathing through the nostrils, inhale steadily, first filling the lower part of the lungs, which is accomplished by bringing into play the diaphragm, which descending exerts a gentle pressure on the abdominal organs, pushing forward the front walls of the abdomen. Then fill the middle part of the lungs, pushing out the lower ribs, breast-bone and chest. Then fill the higher portion of the lungs, protruding the upper chest, thus lifting the chest, including the upper six or seven pairs of ribs. In the final movement, the lower part of the abdomen will be slightly drawn in, which movement gives the lungs a support and also helps to fill the highest part of the lungs.

At first reading it may appear that this breath consists of three distinct movements. This, however, is not the correct idea. The inhalation is continuous, the entire chest cavity from the lowered diaphragm to the highest point of the chest in the region of the collar-bone, being expanded with a uniform movement. Avoid a jerky series of inhalations, and strive to attain a steady continuous action. Practice will soon overcome the tendency to divide the inhalation into three movements, and will result in a uniform continuous breath. You will be able to complete the inhalation in a couple of seconds after a little practice.

(2) Retain the breath a few seconds.

(3) Exhale quite slowly, holding the chest in a firm position, and having the abdomen in a little and lifting it upward slowly as the air leaves the lungs. When the air is entirely exhaled, relax the chest and abdomen. A little practice will render this part of the exercise easy, and the movement once acquired will be afterwards performed almost automatically.

It will be seen that by this method of breathing all parts of the respiratory apparatus is brought into action, and all parts of the lungs, including the most remote air cells, are exercised. The chest cavity is expanded in all directions. You will also notice that the Complete Breath is really a combination of Low, Mid and High Breaths, succeeding each other rapidly in the order given, in such a manner as to form one uniform, continuous, complete breath.

You will find it quite a help to you if you will practice this breath before a large mirror, placing the hands lightly over the abdomen so that you may feel the movements. At the end of the inhalation, it is well to occasionally slightly elevate the shoulders, thus raising the collarbone and allowing the air to pass freely into the small upper lobe of the right lung, which place is sometimes the breeding place of tuberculosis.

At the beginning of practice, you may have more or less trouble in acquiring the Complete Breath, but a little practice will make perfect, and when you have once acquired it you will never willingly return to the old methods.

CHAPTER 9 - PHYSIOLOGICAL EFFECT OF THE COMPLETE BREATH

Scarcely too much can be said of the advantages attending the practice of the Complete Breath. And yet the student who has carefully read the foregoing pages should scarcely need to have pointed out to him such advantages.

The practice of the Complete Breath will make any man or woman immune to Consumption and other pulmonary troubles, and will do away with all liability to contract "colds," as well as bronchial and similar weaknesses. Consumption is due principally to lowered vitality attributable to an insufficient amount of air being inhaled. The impairment of vitality renders the system open to attacks from disease germs. Imperfect breathing allows a considerable part of the lungs to remain inactive, and such portions offer an inviting field for bacilli, which invading the weakened tissue soon produce havoc. Good healthy lung tissue will resist the germs, and the only way to have good healthy lung tissue is to use the lungs properly.

Consumptives are nearly all narrow-chested. What does this mean? Simply that these people were addicted to improper habits of breathing, and consequently their chests failed to develop and expand. The man who practices the Complete Breath will have a full broad chest, end the narrow-chested man may develop his chest to normal proportions if he will but adopt this mode of breathing. Such people must develop their chest cavities if they value their lives. Colds may often be prevented by practicing a little vigorous Complete Breathing whenever you feel that you are being unduly exposed. When chilled, breathe vigorously a few minutes, and you will feel a glow all over your body. Most colds can be cured by Complete Breathing and partial fasting for a day.

The quality of the blood depends largely upon its proper oxygenation in the lungs, and if it is under-oxygenated it becomes poor in quality and laden with all sorts of impurities, and the system suffers from lack of nourishment, and often becomes actually poisoned by the waste products remaining uneliminated in the blood. As the entire body, every organ and every part, is dependent upon the blood for nourishment, impure blood must have a serious effect upon the entire system. The remedy is plain—practice the Yogi Complete Breath.

The stomach and other organs of nutrition suffer much from improper breathing. Not only are they ill nourished by reason of the lack of oxygen, but as the food must absorb oxygen from the blood and become oxygenated before it can be digested and assimilated, it is readily seen how digestion and assimilation is impaired by incorrect breathing. And when assimilation is not normal, the system receives less and less nourishment, the appetite fails, bodily vigor decreases, and energy diminishes, and the man withers and declines. All from the lack of proper breathing.

Even the nervous system suffers from improper breathing, inasmuch as the brain, the spinal cord, the nerve centers, and the nerves themselves, when improperly nourished by means of the blood, become poor and inefficient instruments for generating, storing and transmitting the nerve currents. And improperly nourished they will become if sufficient oxygen is not absorbed through the lungs.

There is another aspect of the case whereby the nerve currents themselves, or rather the force from which the nerve currents spring, becomes lessened from want of proper breathing, but this belongs to another phase of the subject which is treated of in other chapters of this book, and our purpose here is to direct your attention to the fact that the mechanism of the nervous system is rendered inefficient as an instrument for conveying nerve force, as the indirect result of a lack of proper breathing.

The effect of the reproductive organs upon the general health is too well known to be discussed at length here, but we may be permitted to say that with the reproductive organs in a weakened condition the entire system feels the reflex action and suffers sympathetically. The Complete Breath produces a rhythm which is Nature's own plan for keeping this important part of the system in normal condition, and, from the first, it will be noticed that the reproductive functions are strengthened and vitalized, thus, by sympathetic reflex action, giving tone to the whole system. By this, we do not mean that the lower sex impulses will be aroused; far from it. The Yogis are advocates of continence and chastity, and have learned to control the animal passions. But sexual control does not mean sexual weakness, and the Yogi teachings are that the man or woman whose reproductive organism is normal and healthy, will have a stronger will with which to control himself or herself.

The Yogi believes that much of the perversion of this wonderful part of the system comes from a lack of normal health, and results from a morbid rather than a normal condition of these organs. A little careful consideration of this question will prove that the Yogi teachings are right. This is not the place to discuss the subject fully, but the Yogis know that sex-energy may be conserved and used for the development of the body and mind of the individual, instead of being dissipated in unnatural excesses as is the wont of so many uninformed people.

By special request we will give in this book one of the favorite Yogi exercises for this purpose. But whether or not the student wishes to adopt the Yogi theories of continence and clean-living, he or she will find that the Complete Breath will do more to restore health to this part of the system than anything else ever tried. Remember, now, we mean normal health, not undue development. The sensualist will find that normal means a lessening of desire rather than an increase; the weakened man or woman will find a toning up and a relief from the weakness which has heretofore depressed him or her. We do not wish to be misunderstood or misquoted on this subject. The Yogis' ideal is a body strong in all its parts, under the control of a masterful and developed Will, animated by high ideals.

In the practice of the Complete Breath, during inhalation, the diaphragm contracts and exerts a gentle pressure upon the liver, stomach and other organs, which in connection with the rhythm of the lungs acts as a gentle massage of these organs and stimulates their actions, and encourages normal functioning. Each inhalation aids in this internal exercise, and assists in causing a normal circulation to the organs of nutrition and elimination. In High or Mid Breathing the organs lose the benefit accruing from this internal massage.

The Western world is paying much attention to Physical Culture just now, which is a good thing. But in their enthusiasm, they must not forget that the exercise of the external muscles is not everything. The internal organs also need exercise, and Nature's plan for this exercise is proper breathing. The diaphragm is Nature's principal instrument for this internal exercise. Its motion vibrates the important organs of nutrition and elimination, and massages and kneads them at each inhalation and exhalation, forcing blood into them, and then squeezing it out, and imparting a general tone to the organs. Any organ or part of the body which is not exercised gradually atrophies and refuses to function properly, and lack of the internal exercise afforded by the diaphragmatic action leads to diseased organs. The Complete Breath gives the proper motion to the diaphragm, as well as exercising the middle and upper chest. It is indeed "complete" in its action.

From the standpoint of Western physiology alone, without reference to the Oriental philosophies and science, this Yogi system of Complete Breathing is of vital importance to every man, woman and child who wishes to acquire health and keep it. Its very simplicity keeps thousands from seriously considering it, while they spend fortunes in seeking health through complicated and expensive "systems." Health knocks at their door and they answer not. Verily the stone which the builders reject is the real cornerstone of the Temple of Health.

CHAPTER 10 - A FEW BITS OF YOGI LORE

We give below three forms of breath, quite popular among the Yogis. The first is the well-known Yogi Cleansing Breath, to which is attributed much of the great lung endurance found among the Yogis. They usually finish up a breathing exercise with this Cleansing Breath, and we have followed this plan in this book.

We also give the Yogi Nerve Vitalizing Exercise, which has been handed down among them for ages, and which has never been improved on by Western teachers of Physical Culture, although some of them have "borrowed" it from teachers of Yoga. We also give the Yogi Vocal Breath, which accounts largely for the melodious, vibrant voices of the better class of the Oriental Yogis. We feel that if this book contained nothing more than these three exercises, it would be invaluable to the Western student. Take these exercises as a gift from your Eastern brothers and put them into practice.

THE YOGI CLEANSING BREATH

The Yogis have a favorite form of breathing which they practice when they feel the necessity of ventilating and cleansing the lungs. They conclude many of their other breathing exercises with this breath, and we have followed this practice in this book. This Cleansing Breath ventilates and cleanses the lungs, stimulates the cells and gives a general tone to the respiratory organs, and is conducive to their general healthy condition. Besides this effect, it is found to greatly refresh the entire system. Speakers, singers, etc., will find this breath especially restful, after having tired the respiratory organs.

(1) Inhale a complete breath.

(2) Retain the air a few seconds.

(3) Pucker up the lips as if for a whistle (but do not swell out the cheeks), then exhale a little air through the opening, with considerable vigor. Then stop for a moment, retaining the air, and then exhale a little more air. Repeat until the air is completely exhaled. Remember that considerable vigor is to be used in exhaling the air through the opening in the lips.

This breath will be found quite refreshing when one is tired and generally "used up." A trial will convince the student of its merits. This exercise should be practiced until it can be performed naturally and easily, as it is used to finish up a number of other exercises given in this book, and it should be thoroughly understood.

THE YOGI NERVE VITALIZING BREATH

This is an exercise well known to the Yogis, who consider it one of the strongest nerve stimulants and invigorants known to man. Its purpose is to stimulate the Nervous System, develop nerve force, energy and vitality. This exercise brings a stimulating pressure to bear on important nerve centers, which in turn stimulate and energize the entire nervous system, and send an increased flow of nerve force to all parts of the body.

(1) Stand erect.

(2) Inhale a Complete Breath, and retain same.

(3) Extend the arms straight in front of you, letting them be somewhat limp and relaxed, with only sufficient nerve force to hold them out.

(4) Slowly draw the hands back toward the shoulders, gradually contracting the muscles and putting force into them, so that when they reach the shoulders the fists will be so tightly clenched that a tremulous motion is felt.

(5) Then, keeping the muscles tense, push the fists slowly out, and then draw them back rapidly (still tense) several times.

(6) Exhale vigorously through the mouth.

(7) Practice the Cleansing Breath.

The efficiency of this exercise depends greatly upon the speed of the drawing back of the fists, and the tension of the muscles, and, of course, upon the full lungs. This exercise must be tried to be appreciated. It is without equal as a "bracer," as our Western friends put it.

THE YOGI VOCAL BREATH

The Yogis have a form of breathing to develop the voice. They are noted for their wonderful voices, which are strong, smooth and clear, and have a wonderful trumpet-like carrying power. They have practiced this particular form of breathing exercise which has resulted in rendering their voices soft, beautiful and flexible, imparting to it that indescribable, peculiar floating quality, combined with great power. The exercise given below will in time impart the above-mentioned qualities, or the Yogi Voice, to the student who practices it faithfully. It is to be understood, of course, that this form of breath is to be used only as an occasional exercise, and not as a regular form of breathing.

(1) Inhale a Complete Breath very slowly, but steadily, through the nostrils, taking as much time as possible in the inhalation.

(2) Retain for a few seconds.

(3) Expel the air vigorously in one great breath, through the wide opened mouth.

(4) Rest the lungs by the Cleansing Breath.

Without going deeply into the Yogi theories of sound-production in speaking and singing, we wish to say that experience has taught them that the timbre, quality and power of a voice depends not alone upon the vocal organs in the throat, but that the facial muscles, etc., have much to do with the matter. Some men with large chests produce but a poor tone, while others with comparatively small chests produce tones of amazing strength and quality. Here is an interesting experiment worth trying: Stand before a glass and pucker up your mouth and whistle, and note the shape of your mouth and the general expression of your face. Then sing or speak as you do naturally, and see the difference. Then start to whistle again for a few seconds, and then, *without changing the position of your lips or face*, sing a few notes and notice what a vibrant, resonant, clear and beautiful tone is produced.

CHAPTER 11 - THE SEVEN YOGI DEVELOPING EXERCISES

The following are the seven favorite exercises of the Yogis for developing the lungs, muscles, ligaments, air cells, etc. They are quite simple but marvelously effective.

Do not let the simplicity of these exercises make you lose interest, for they are the result of careful experiments and practice on the part of the Yogis, and are the essence of numerous intricate and complicated exercises, the non-essential portions being eliminated and the essential features retained.

THE RETAINED BREATH

This is a very important exercise which tends to strengthen and develop the respiratory muscles as well as the lungs, and its frequent practice will also tend to expand the chest. The Yogis have found that an occasional holding of the breath, after the lungs have been filled with the Complete Breath, is very beneficial, not only to the respiratory organs but to the organs of nutrition, the nervous system and the blood itself. They have found that an occasional holding of the breath tends to purify the air which has remained in the lungs from former inhalations, and to more fully oxygenate the blood.

They also know that the breath so retained gathers up all the waste matter, and when the breath is expelled it carries with it the effete matter of the system, and cleanses the lungs just as a purgative does the bowels. The Yogis recommend this exercise for various disorders of the stomach, liver and blood, and also find that it frequently relieves bad breath, which often arises from poorly ventilated lungs. We recommend students to pay considerable attention to this exercise, as it has great merits.

The following directions will give you a clear idea of the exercise:

1. Stand erect.
2. Inhale a Complete Breath.
3. Retain the air as long as you can comfortably.
4. Exhale vigorously through the open mouth.
5. Practice the Cleansing Breath.

At first you will be able to retain the breath only a short time, but a little practice will also show a great improvement. Time yourself with a watch if you wish to note your progress.

LUNG CELL STIMULATION

This exercise is designed to stimulate the air cells in the lungs, but beginners must not overdo it, and in no case should it be indulged in too vigorously. Some may find a slight dizziness resulting from the first few trials, in which case let them walk around a little and discontinue the exercise for a while.

1. Stand erect, with hands at sides.
2. Breathe in very slowly and gradually.
3. While inhaling, gently tap the chest with the finger tips, constantly changing position.
4. When the lungs are filled, retain the breath and pat the chest with the palms of the hands.
5. Practice the Cleansing Breath.

This exercise is very bracing and stimulating to the whole body, and is a well-known Yogi practice. Many of the air cells of the lungs become inactive by reason of incomplete breathing, and often become almost atrophied. One who has practiced imperfect breathing for years will find it not so easy to stimulate all these ill-used air cells into activity all at once by the Complete Breath, but this exercise will do much toward bringing about the desired result, and is worth study and practice.

RIB STRETCHING

We have explained that the ribs are fastened by cartilages, which admit of considerable expansion. In proper breathing, the ribs play an important part, and it is well to occasionally give them a little special exercise in order to preserve their elasticity. Standing or sitting in unnatural positions, to which many of the Western people are addicted, is apt to render the ribs more or less stiff and inelastic, and this exercise will do much to overcome same.

1. Stand erect.
2. Place the hands one on each side of the body, as high up under the armpits as convenient, the thumbs reaching toward the back, the palms on the side of the chest and the fingers to the front over the breast.
3. Inhale a Complete Breath.
4. Retain the air for a short time.
5. Then gently squeeze the sides, at the same time slowly exhaling.
6. Practice the cleansing breath.

Use moderation in this exercise and do not overdo its

CHEST EXPANSION

The chest is quite apt to be contracted from bending over one's work, etc. This exercise is very good for the purpose of restoring natural conditions and gaining chest expansion.

1. Stand erect.
2. Inhale a Complete Breath.
3. Retain the air.
4. Extend both arms forward and bring the two clenched fists together on a level with the shoulder.
5. Then swing back the fists vigorously until the arms stand out straight sideways from the shoulders.
6. Then bring back to Position 4, and swing to Position 5. Repeat several times.
7. Exhale vigorously through the opened mouth.
8. Practice the Cleansing Breath.

Use moderation and do not overdo this exercise.

WALKING EXERCISE

1. Walk with head up, chin drawn slightly in, shoulders back, and with measured tread.
2. Inhale a Complete Breath, counting (mentally) 1, 2, 3, 4, 5, 6, 7, 8, one count to each step, making the inhalation extend over the eight counts.
3. Exhale slowly through the nostrils, counting as before—1, 2, 3, 4, 5, 6, 7, 8—one count to a step.
4. Rest between breaths, continuing walking and counting, I, 2, 3, 4, 5, 8, 7, 8, one count to a step.
5. Repeat until you begin to feel tired. Then rest for a while, and resume at pleasure. Repeat several times a day.

Some Yogis vary this exercise by retaining the breath during a 1, 2, 3, 4, count, and then exhale in an eight-step count. Practice whichever plan seems most agreeable to you.

MORNING EXERCISE

1. Stand erect in a military attitude, head up, eyes front, shoulders back, knees stiff, hands at sides.

2. Raise body slowly on toes, inhaling a Complete Breath, steadily and slowly.
3. Retain the breath for a few seconds, maintaining the same position.
4. Slowly sink to first position, at the same time slowly exhaling the air through the nostrils.
5. Practice Cleansing Breath.
6. Repeat several times, varying by using right leg alone, then left leg alone.

STIMULATING CIRCULATION

1. Stand erect.
2. Inhale a Complete Breath and retain.
3. Bend forward slightly and grasp a stick or cane steadily and firmly, and gradually exerting your entire strength upon the grasp.
4. Relax the grasp, return to first position, and slowly exhale.
5. Repeat several times.
6. Finish with the Cleansing Breath.

This exercise may be performed without the use of a stick or cane, by grasping an imaginary cane, using the will to exert the pressure. The exercise is a favorite Yogi plan of stimulating the circulation by driving the arterial blood to the extremities, and drawing back the venous blood to the heart and lungs that it may take up the oxygen which has been inhaled with the air. In cases of poor circulation there is not enough blood in the lungs to absorb the increased amount of oxygen inhaled, and the system does not get the full benefit of the improved breathing.

In such cases, particularly, It Is well to practice this exercise, occasionally with the regular Complete Breathing exercise.

CHAPTER 12 - SEVEN MINOR YOGI EXERCISES

This chapter is composed of seven minor Yogi Breathing Exercises, bearing no special names, but each distinct and separate from the others and having a different purpose in view. Each student will find several of these exercises best adapted to the special requirements of his particular case. Although we have styled these exercises "minor exercises," they are quite valuable and useful, or they would not appear in this book. They give one a condensed course in "Physical Culture" and "Lung Development," and might readily be "padded out" and elaborated into a small book on these subjects. They have, of course, an additional value, as Yogi Breathing forms a part of each exercise. Do not pass them by because they are marked "minor." Some one or more of these exercises may be just what you need. Try them and decide for yourself.

EXERCISE 1

1. Stand erect with hands at sides.
2. Inhale Complete Breath.
3. Raise the arms slowly, keeping them rigid until the hands touch overhead.
4. Retain the breath a few minutes with hands over head.
5. Lower hands slowly to sides, exhaling slowly at same time.
6. Practice Cleansing Breath.

EXERCISE 2

1. Stand erect, with arms straight In front of you.
2. Inhale Complete Breath and retain.
3. Swing arms back as far as they will go; then back to first position; then repeat several times, returning the breath all the while.
4. Exhale vigorously through mouth.
5. Practice Cleansing Breath.

EXERCISE 3

1. Stand erect with arms straight In front of you,
2. Inhale Complete Breath.
3. Swing arms around in a circle, backward, a few times. Then reverse a few times, retaining the breath all the while. You may vary this by rotating them alternately like the sails of a windmill.
4. Exhale the breath vigorously through the mouth.

5. Practice Cleansing Breath.

EXERCISE 4

1. Lie on the floor with your face downward and palms of hands flat upon the floor by your sides.
2. Inhale Complete Breath and retain.
3. Stiffen the body and raise yourself up by the strength of your arms until you rest on your hands and toes
4. Then lower yourself to original position. Repeat several times.
5. Exhale vigorously through your mouth.
6. Practice Cleansing Breath.

EXERCISE 5

1. Stand erect with your palms against the wall.
2. Inhale Complete Breath and retain.
3. Lower the chest to the wall, resting your weight on your hands.
4. Then raise yourself back with the arm muscles alone, keeping the body stiff.
5. Exhale vigorously through the mouth.
6. Practice Cleansing Breath.

EXERCISE 6

1. Stand erect with arms "akimbo," that is, with hands resting around the waist and elbows standing out.
2. Inhale Complete Breath and retain.
3. Keep legs and hips stiff and bend well forward, as If bowing, at the same time exhaling slowly.
4. Return to first position and take another Complete Breath.
5. Then bend backward, exhaling slowly.
6. Return to first position and take a Complete Breath.
7. Then bend sideways, exhaling slowly. (Vary by bending to right and then to left.)
8. Practice Cleansing Breath.

EXERCISE 7

1. Stand erect, or sit erect, with straight spinal column.

2. Inhale a Complete Breath, but instead of inhaling in a continuous steady stream, take a series of short, quick "sniffs," as if you were smelling aromatic salts or ammonia and did not wish to get too strong a "whiff." Do not exhale any of these little breaths, but add one to the other until the entire lung space Is filled.
3. Retain for a few seconds.
4. Exhale through the nostrils in a long, restful, sighing breath.
5. Practice Cleansing Breath.

CHAPTER 13 - VIBRATION AND YOGI RHYTHMIC BREATHING

All is in vibration. From the tiniest atom to the greatest sun, everything is in a state of vibration. There is nothing in absolute rest in nature. A single atom deprived of vibration would wreck the universe. In incessant vibration the universal work is performed. Matter is being constantly played upon by energy and countless forms and numberless varieties result, and yet even the forms and varieties are not permanent. They begin to change the moment they are created, and from them are born innumerable forms, which in turn change and give rise to newer forms, and so on and on, in infinite succession. Nothing is permanent in the world of forms, and yet the great Reality is unchangeable. Forms are but appearances—they come, they go, but the Reality is eternal and unchangeable.

The atoms of the human body are in constant vibration. Unceasing changes are occurring. In a few months there is almost a complete change in the matter composing the body, and scarcely a single atom now composing your body will be found in It a few months hence. Vibration, constant vibration. Change, constant change.

In all vibration is to be found a certain rhythm. Rhythm pervades the universe. The swing of the planets around the sun; the rise and fall of the sea; the beating of the heart; the ebb and flow of the tide; all follow rhythmics laws. The rays of the sun reach us; the rain descends upon us, in obedience to the same law. All growth is but an exhibition of this law. All motion is a manifestation of the law of rhythm.

Our bodies are as much subject to rhythmic laws as is the planet in its revolution around the sun. Much of the esoteric side of the Yogi Science of Breath is based upon this known principle of nature. By falling in with the rhythm of the body, the Yogi manages to absorb a great amount of Prana, which he disposes of to bring about results desired by him. We will speak of this at greater length later on.

The body which you occupy is like a small inlet running in to the land from the sea. Although apparently subject only to its own laws, it is really subject to the ebb and flow of the tides of the ocean. The great sea of life is swelling and receding, rising and falling, and we are responding to its vibrations and rhythm. In a normal condition we receive the vibration and rhythm of the great ocean of life, and respond to it, but at times the mouth of the inlet seems choked up with debris, and we fail to receive the impulse from Mother Ocean, and inharmony manifests within us.

You have heard how a note on a violin, if sounded repeatedly and in rhythm, will start into motion vibrations which will in time destroy a bridge. The same result is true when a regiment of soldiers crosses a bridge, the order being always given to "break step" on such an occasion, lest the vibration bring down both bridge and regiment. These manifestations of the effect of rhythmic motion will give you an idea of the effect on the body of rhythmic breathing.

The whole system catches the vibration and becomes in harmony with the will, which causes the rhythmic motion of the lungs, and while in such complete harmony will respond readily to orders from the will. With the body thus attuned, the Yogi finds no difficulty in increasing the circulation in any part of the body by an order from the will, and in the same way he can direct an increased current of nerve force to any part or organ, strengthening and stimulating it.

In the same way the Yogi by rhythmic breathing "catches the swing," as it were, and is able to absorb and control a greatly increased amount of prana, which is then at the disposal of his will. He can and does use it as a vehicle for sending forth thoughts to others and for attracting to him all those whose thoughts are keyed in the same vibration. The phenomena of telepathy, thought transference, mental healing, mesmerism, etc., which subjects are creating such an interest in the Western world at the present time, but which have been known to the Yogis for centuries, can be greatly increased and augmented If the person sending forth the thoughts will do so after rhythmic breathing. Rhythmic breathing will increase the value of mental healing, magnetic healing, etc., several hundred per cent.

In rhythmic breathing the main thing to be acquired is the mental idea of rhythm. To those who know anything of music, the idea of measured counting is familiar. To others, the rhythmic step of the soldier: "Left, right; left, right; left, right; one, two, three, four; one, two, three, four," will convey the idea.

The Yogi bases his rhythmic time upon a unit corresponding with the beat of his heart. The heart beat varies in different persons, but the heart beat unit of each person is the proper rhythmic standard for that particular individual in his rhythmic breathing. Ascertain your normal heart beat by placing your fingers over your pulse, and then count: "1, 2, 3, 4, 5, 6; 1, 2, 3, 4, 5, 6," etc., until the rhythm becomes firmly fixed in your mind. A little practice will fix the rhythm, so that you will be able to easily reproduce it. The beginner usually inhales in about six pulse units, but he will be able to greatly increase this by practice.

The Yogi rule for rhythmic breathing is that the units of inhalation and exhalation should be the same, while the units for retention and between breaths should be one-half the number of those of inhalation and exhalation.

The following exercise in Rhythmic Breathing should be thoroughly mastered, as it forms the basis of numerous other exercises, to which reference will be made later.

1. Sit erect, in an easy posture, being sure to hold the chest, neck and head as nearly in a straight line as possible, with shoulders slightly thrown back and hands resting easily on the lap. In this position the weight of the body is largely supported by the ribs and the position may be easily maintained. The Yogi has found that one cannot get the best effect of rhythmic breathing with the chest drawn in and the abdomen protruding.
2. Inhale slowly a Complete Breath, counting six pulse units.
3. Retain, counting three pulse units.
4. Exhale slowly through the nostrils, counting six pulse units.
5. Count three pulse beats between breaths.
6. Repeat a number of times, but avoid fatiguing yourself at the start.
7. When you are ready to close the exercise, practice the cleansing breath, which will rest you and cleanse the lungs.

After a little practice you will be able to increase the duration of the inhalations and exhalations, until about fifteen pulse units are consumed. In this increase, remember that the units for retention and between breaths is one-half the units for inhalation and exhalation.

Do not overdo yourself in your effort to increase the duration of the breath, but pay as much attention as possible to acquiring the "rhythm," as that is more important than the length of the breath. Practice and try until you get the measured "swing" of the movement, and until you can almost "feel" the rhythm of the vibratory motion throughout your whole body. It will require a little practice and perseverance, but your pleasure at your improvement will make the task an easy one. The Yogi is a most patient and persevering man, and his great attainments are due largely to the possession of these qualities.

CHAPTER 14 - PHENOMENA OF YOGI PSYCHIC BREATHING

With the exception of the instructions in the Yogi Rhythmic Breathing, the majority of the exercises heretofore given in this book relate to the physical plane of effort, which, while highly important in itself, is also regarded by the Yogis as in the nature of affording a substantial basis for efforts on the psychic and spiritual plane. Do not, however, discard or think lightly of the physical phase of the subject, for remember that it needs a sound body to support a sound mind, and also that the body is the temple of the Ego, the lamp in which burns the light of the Spirit. Everything is good in its place, and everything has its place. The developed man is the "all-around man," who recognizes body, mind and spirit and renders to each its due. Neglect of either is a mistake which must be rectified sooner or later; a debt which must be repaid with interest.

We will now take up the Psychic phase of the Yogi Science of Breath in the shape of a series of exercises, each exercise carrying with it its explanation.

You will notice that in each exercise rhythmic breathing is accompanied with the instructions to "carry the thought" of certain desired results. This mental attitude gives the Will a cleared track upon which to exercise its force. We cannot, in this work, go into the subject of the power of the Will, and must assume that you have some knowledge of the subject. If you have no acquaintance with the subject, you will find that the actual practice of the exercises themselves will give you a much clearer knowledge than any amount of theoretical teaching, for as the old Hindu proverb says, "He who tastes a grain of mustard seed knows more of its flavor than he who sees an elephant load of it."

GENERAL DIRECTIONS FOR YOGI PSYCHIC BREATHING

The basis of all Yogi Psychic Breathing is the Yogi Rhythmic Breath, instruction regarding which we gave in our last chapter. In the following exercises, in order to avoid useless repetition, we will say merely, "Breathe Rhythmically," and then give the instruction for the exercise of the psychic force, or directed Will power working in connection with the rhythmic breath vibrations. After a little practice you will find that you will not need to count after the first rhythmic breath, as the mind will grasp the idea of time and rhythm and you will be able to breathe rhythmically at pleasure, almost automatically. This will leave the mind clear for the sending of the psychic vibrations under the direction of the Will. (See the following first exercise for directions in using the Will.)

PRANA DISTRIBUTING

Lying flat on the floor or bed, completely relaxed, with hands resting lightly over the Solar Plexus (over the pit of the stomach, where the ribs begin to separate), breathe rhythmically. After the rhythm is fully established *will* that each inhalation will draw in an increased supply of prana or vital energy from the Universal supply, which will be taken up by the nervous system and stored in the Solar Plexus. At each exhalation will that the prana or vital energy is being distributed all over the body, to every organ and part; to every muscle, cell and atom; to nerve, artery and vein; from the top of your head to the soles of your feet; invigorating, strengthening and stimulating every nerve; recharging every nerve center; sending energy, force and strength all over the system. While exercising the will, try to form a mental picture of the inrushing prana, coming in through the lungs and being taken up at once by the Solar Plexus, then with the exhaling effort, being sent to all parts of the system, down to the finger tips and down to the toes. It is not necessary to use the Will with an effort. Simply commanding that which you wish to produce and then making the mental picture of it is all that is necessary. Calm command with the mental picture is far better than forcible willing, which only dissipates force needlessly. The above exercise is most helpful and greatly refreshes and strengthens the nervous system and produces a restful feeling all over the body. It is especially beneficial In cases where one is tired or feels a lack of energy.

INHIBITING PAIN

Lying down or sitting erect, breath rhythmically, holding the thought that you are inhaling prana. Then when you exhale, send the prana to the painful part to re-establish the circulation and nerve current. Then inhale more prana for the purpose of driving out the painful condition; then exhale, holding the thought that you are driving out the pain. Alternate the two above mental commands, and with one exhalation stimulate the part and with the next drive out the pain. Keep this up for seven breaths, then practice the Cleansing Breath and rest a while. Then try it again until relief comes, which will be before long. Many pains will be found to be relieved before the seven breaths are finished. If the hand is placed over the painful part, you may get quicker results. Send the current of prana down the arm and into the painful part.

DIRECTING THE CIRCULATION

Lying down or sitting erect, breathe rhythmically, and with the exhalations direct the circulation to any part you wish, which may be suffering from imperfect circulation. This is effective in cases of cold feet or in cases of headache, the blood being sent downward in both cases, in the first case warming the feet, and in the latter, relieving the brain from too great pressure. In the case of headache, try the Pain Inhibiting first, then follow with sending the blood downward. You will often feel a warm feeling in the legs as the circulation moves downward. The circulation is largely under the control of the will and rhythmic breathing renders the task easier.

SELF-HEALING

Lying in a relaxed condition, breathe rhythmically, and command that a good supply of prana be inhaled. With the exhalation, send the prana to the affected part for the purpose of stimulating it. Vary this occasionally by exhaling, with the mental command that the diseased condition be forced out and disappear. Use the hands in this exercise, passing them down the body from the head to the affected part. In using the hands in healing yourself or others, always hold the mental image that the prana is flowing down the arm and through the finger tips into the body, thus reaching the affected part and healing it.

Of course, we can give only general directions in this book without taking up the several forms of disease in detail, but a little practice of the above exercise, varying it slightly to fit the conditions of the case, will produce wonderful results. Some Yogis follow the plan of placing both hands on the affected part, and then breathing rhythmically, holding the mental image that they are fairly pumping prana into the diseased organ and part, stimulating it and driving out diseased conditions, as pumping into a pail of dirty water will drive out the latter and fill the bucket with fresh water. This last plan is very effective if the mental image of the pump is clearly held, the inhalation representing the lifting of the pump handle and the exhalation the actual pumping.

HEALING OTHERS

We cannot take up the question of the psychic treatment of disease by prana in detail in this book, as such would be foreign to its purpose. But we can and will give you simple, plain instructions whereby you may be enabled to do much good in relieving others. The main principle to remember is that by rhythmic breathing and controlled thought you are enabled to absorb a considerable amount of prana, and are also able to pass it into the body of another person, stimulating weakened parts and organs and imparting health and driving out diseased conditions. You must first learn to form such a clear mental image of the desired condition that you will be able to actually feel the influx of prana, and the force running down your arms and out of your fingertips into the body of the patient. Breathe rhythmically a few times until the rhythm is fairly established, then place your bands upon the affected part of the body of the patient, letting them rest lightly over the part. Then follow the "pumping" process described to the preceding exercise (Self-Healing) and fill the patient full of prana until the diseased condition is driven out.

Every once in a while, raise the hands and "flick" the fingers as if you were throwing off the diseased condition. It is well to do this occasionally and also to wash the hands after treatment, as otherwise you may take on a trace of the diseased condition of the patient. Also practice the Cleansing Breath several times after the treatment.

During the treatment let the prana pour into the patient in one continuous stream, allowing yourself to be merely the pumping machinery connecting the patient with the universal supply of prana, and allowing it to flow freely through you. You need not work the hands vigorously, but simply enough that the prana freely reaches the affected parts.

The rhythmic breathing must be practiced frequently during the treatment, so as to keep the rhythm normal and to afford the prana a free passage. It is better to place the hands on the bare skin, but where this is not advisable or possible place them over the clothing. Vary above method occasionally during the treatment by stroking the body gently and softly with the finger tips, the fingers being kept slightly separated. This is very soothing to the patient. In cases of long standing, you may find it helpful to give the mental command in words, such as "get out, get out," or "be strong, be strong," as the case may be, the words helping you to exercise the will more forcibly and to the point.

Vary these instructions to suit the needs of the case, and use your own judgment and inventive faculty. We have given you the general principles and you can apply them in hundreds of different ways. The above apparently simple instruction, if carefully studied and applied, will enable one to accomplish all that the leading "magnetic healers" are able to, although their "systems" are more or less cumbersome and complicated. They are using prana ignorantly and calling it "magnetism." If they would combine rhythmic breathing with their "magnetic" treatment they would double their efficiency.

DISTANT HEALING

Prana colored by the thought of the sender may be projected to persons at a distance, who are willing to receive it, and healing work done in this way. This is the secret of the "absent healing," of which the Western world has heard so much of late years. The thought of the healer sends forth and colors the prana of the sender, and it flashes across space and finds lodgment in the psychic mechanism of the patient. It is unseen, and like the Marconi waves, it passes through intervening obstacles and seeks the person attuned to receive it. In order to treat persons at a distance, you must form a mental image of them until you can feel yourself to be in rapport with them. This is a psychic process dependent upon the mental imagery of the healer.

You can feel the sense of rapport when it is established, it manifesting in a sense of nearness. That is about as plain as we can describe it. It may be acquired by a little practice, and some will get it at the first trial. When rapport is established, say mentally to the distant patient, "I am sending you a supply of vital force or power, which will invigorate you and heal you." Then picture the prana as leaving your mind with each exhalation of rhythmic breath, and traveling across space instantaneously and reaching the patient and healing him. It is not necessary to fix certain hours for treatment, although you may do so if you wish.

The receptive condition of the patient, as he is expecting and opening himself up to your psychic force, attunes him to receive your vibrations whenever you may send them. If you agree upon hours, let him place himself in a relaxed attitude and receptive condition. The above is the great underlying principle of the "absent treatment" of the Western world. You may do these things as well as the most noted healers, with a little practice.

CHAPTER 15 - MORE PHENOMENA OF YOGI PSYCHIC BREATHING

THOUGHT PROJECTION

Thoughts may be projected by following the last-mentioned method (Distant Healing) and others will feel the effect of thought so sent forth, it being remembered always that no evil thought can ever injure another person whose thoughts are good. Good thoughts are always positive to bad ones, and bad ones always negative to good ones. One can, however, excite the interest and attention of another by sending him thought waves in this way, charging the prana with the message he wishes to convey.

If you desire another's love and sympathy, and possess love and sympathy for him, you can send him thoughts of this kind with effect, providing your motives are pure. Never, however, attempt to influence another to his hurt, or from impure or selfish motives, as such thoughts only recoil upon the sender with redoubled force, and injure him, while the innocent party is not affected. Psychic force when legitimately used is all right, but beware of "black magic" or improper and unholy uses of it, as such attempts are like playing with a dynamo, and the person attempting such things will be surely punished by the result of the act itself. However, no person of impure motives ever acquires a great degree of psychic power, and a pure heart and mind is an invulnerable shield against improper psychic power. Keep yourself pure and nothing can hurt you.

FORMING AN AURA

If you are ever in the company of persons of a low order of mind, and you feel the depressing influence of their thought, breathe rhythmically a few times, thus generating an additional supply of prana, and then by means of the mental image method surround yourself with an egg-shaped thought aura, which will protect you from the gross thought and disturbing influences of others.

RECHARGING YOURSELF

If you feel that your vital energy is at a low ebb, and that you need to store up a new supply quickly, the best plan is to place the feet close together (side by side, of course) and to lock the fingers of both hands in any way that seems the most comfortable. This closes the circuit, as it were, and prevents any escape of prana through the extremities. Then breathe rhythmically a few times, and you will feel the effect of the recharging.

RECHARGING OTHERS

If some friend is deficient in vitality you may aid him by sitting in front of him, your toes touching his, and his hands in yours. Then both breathe rhythmically, you forming the mental image of sending prana into his system, and he holding the mental image of receiving the prana. Persons of weak vitality or passive will should be careful with whom they try this experiment, as the prana of a person of evil desires will be colored with the thoughts of that person, and may give him a temporary influence over the weaker person. The latter, however, may easily remove such influence by closing the circuit (as before mentioned) and breathing a few rhythmic breaths, closing with the Cleansing Breath.

CHARGING WATER

Water may be charged with prana, by breathing rhythmically, and holding the glass of water by the bottom, in the left hand, and then gathering the fingers of the right hand together and shaking them gently over the water, as if you were shaking drops of water off of your fingertips into the glass. The mental image of the prana being passed into the water must also be held. Water thus charged is found stimulating to weak or sick persons, particularly if a healing thought accompanies the mental image of the transfer of the prana. The caution given in the last exercise applies also to this one, although the danger exists only in a greatly lessened degree.

ACQUIRING MENTAL QUALITIES

Not only can the body be controlled by the mind under direction of the will, but the mind itself can be trained and cultivated by the exercise of the controlling will. This, which the Western world knows as "Mental Science," etc., has proved to the West portions of that truth which the Yogi has known for ages. The mere calm demand of the Will will accomplish wonders in this direction, but if the mental exercise is accompanied by rhythmic breathing, the effect is greatly increased. Desirable qualities may be acquired by holding the proper mental image of what is desired during rhythmic breathing. Poise and Self Control, desirable qualities; increased power, etc., may be acquired in this way. Undesirable qualities may be eliminated by cultivating the opposite qualities. Any or all the "Mental Science" exercises, "treatments" and "affirmations" may be used with the Yogi Rhythmic

Breath. The following is a good general exercise for the acquirement and development of desirable mental qualities:

Lie in a passive attitude, or sit erect. Picture to yourself the qualities you desire to cultivate, seeing yourself as possessed of the qualities, and demanding that your mind develop the quality. Breathe rhythmically, holding the mental picture firmly. Carry the mental picture with you as much as possible, and endeavor to live up to the ideal you have set up in your mind. You will find yourself gradually growing up to your ideal. The rhythm of the breathing assists the mind in forming new combinations, and the student who has followed the Western system will find the Yogi Rhythmic a wonderful ally in his "Mental Science" works.

ACQUIRING PHYSICAL QUALITIES

Physical qualities may be acquired by the same methods as above mentioned in connection with mental qualities. We do not mean, of course, that short men can be made tall, or that amputated limbs may be replaced, or similar miracles. But the expression of the countenance may be changed; courage and general physical characteristics improved by the control of the Will, accompanied by rhythmic breathing. As a man thinks so does he look, act, walk, sit, etc. Improved thinking will mean improved looks and actions. To develop any part of the body, direct the attention to it, while breathing rhythmically, holding the mental picture that you are sending an increased amount of prana, or nerve force, to the part, and thus increasing its vitality and developing it. This plan applies equally well to any part of the body which you wish to develop. Many Western athletes use a modification of this plan in their exercises. The student who has followed our instructions so far will readily understand how to apply the Yogi principles in the above work. The general rule of exercise is the same as in the preceding exercise (acquiring Mental Qualities). We have touched upon the subject of the cure of physical ailments in preceding pages.

CONTROLLING THE EMOTIONS

The undesirable emotions, such as Fear, Worry, Anxiety, Hate, Anger, Jealousy, Envy, Melancholy, Excitement, Grief, etc., are amenable to the control of the Will, and the Will is enabled to operate more easily in such cases if rhythmic breathing is practiced while the student is "willing." The following exercise has been found most effective by the Yogi students, although the advanced Yogi has but little need of it, as he has long since gotten rid of these undesirable mental qualities by growing spiritually beyond them. The Yogi student, however, finds the exercise a great help to him while he is growing.

Breathe rhythmically, concentrating the attention upon the Solar Plexus, and sending to it the mental command "Get Out." Send the mental command firmly, just as you begin to exhale, and form the mental picture of the undesirable emotions being carried away with the exhaled breath. Repeat seven times, and finish with the Cleansing Breath, and then see how good you feel. The mental command must be given "in earnest," as trifling will not do the work.

TRANSMUTATION OF THE REPRODUCTIVE ENERGY

The Yogis possess great knowledge regarding the use and abuse of the reproductive principle in both sexes. Some hints of this esoteric knowledge have filtered out and have been used by Western writers on the subject, and much good has been accomplished in this way. In this little book we cannot do more than touch upon the subject, and omitting all except a bare mention of theory, we will give a practical breathing exercise whereby the student will be enabled to transmute the reproductive energy into vitality for the entire system, instead of dissipating and wasting it in lustful indulgences in or out of the marriage relations. The reproductive energy is creative energy, and may be taken up by the system and transmuted into strength and vitality, thus serving the purpose of regeneration instead of generation. If the young men of the Western world understood these underlying principles, they would be saved much misery and unhappiness in after years, and would be stronger mentally, morally and physically.

This transmutation of the reproductive energy gives great vitality to those practicing it. They will be filled with great vital force, which will radiate from them and will manifest in what has been called "personal magnetism." The energy thus transmuted may be turned into new channels and used to great advantage. Nature has condensed one of its most powerful manifestations of prana into reproductive energy, as its purpose is to create. The greatest amount of vital force is concentrated in the smallest area. The reproductive organism is the most powerful storage battery in animal life, and its force can be drawn upward and used, as well as expended in the ordinary functions of reproduction, or wasted in riotous lust. The majority of our students know something of the theories of regeneration; and we can do little more than to state the above facts, without attempting to prove them.

The Yogi exercise for transmuting reproductive energy is simple. It is coupled with rhythmic breathing, and can be easily performed. It may be practiced at any time, but is specially recommended when one feels the instinct most strongly, at which time the reproductive energy is manifesting and may be most easily transmuted for regenerative purposes. The exercise is as follows: Keep the mind fixed on the idea of Energy, and away from ordinary sexual thoughts or imaginings.

If these thoughts come into the mind do not be discouraged, but regard them as manifestations of a force which you intend using for the purposes of strengthening the body and mind. Lie passively or sit erect, and fix your mind on the idea of drawing the reproductive energy upward to the Solar Plexus, where it will be transmuted and stored away as a reserve force of vital energy. Then breathe rhythmically, forming the mental image of drawing up the reproductive energy with each inhalation. With each inhalation make a command of the Will that the energy be drawn upward from the reproductive organization to the Solar Plexus. If the rhythm is fairly established and the mental image is clear, you will be conscious of the upward passage of the energy, and will feel its stimulating effect. If you desire an increase in mental force, you may draw it up to the brain instead of to the Solar Plexus, by giving the mental command and holding the mental image of the transmission to the brain.

The man or woman doing metal creative work, or bodily creative work, will be able to use this creative energy in their work by following the above exercise, drawing up the energy with the inhalation and sending it forth with the exhalation. In this last form of exercise, only such portions as are needed in the work will pass into the work being done, the balance remaining stored up in the Solar Plexus. You will understand, of course, that it is not the reproductive fluids which are drawn up and used, but the etheripranic energy which animates the latter, the soul of the reproductive organism, as it were. It is usual to allow the head to bend forward easily and naturally during the transmuting exercise.

BRAIN STIMULATING

The Yogis have found the following exercise most useful in stimulating the action of the brain for the purpose of producing clear thinking and reasoning. It has a wonderful effect in clearing the brain and nervous system, and those engaged in mental work will find it most useful to them, both in the direction of enabling them to do better work and also as a means of refreshing the mind and clearing it after arduous mental labor.

Sit in an erect posture, keeping the spinal column straight, and the eyes well to the front, letting the hands rest on the upper part of the legs. Breathe rhythmically, but instead of breathing through both nostrils as in the ordinary exercises, press the left nostril close with the thumb, and inhale through the right nostril. Then remove the thumb, and close the right nostril with the finger, and then exhale through the left nostril. Then, without changing the fingers, inhale through the left nostril, and changing fingers, exhale through the right. Then inhale through right and exhale through left, and so on, alternating nostrils as above mentioned, closing the unused nostril with the thumb or forefinger. This is one of the oldest forms of Yogi breathing, and is quite important and valuable, and is well worthy of acquirement. But it is quite amusing to the Yogis to know that to the Western world this method is often held out as being the "whole secret" of Yogi Breathing. To the minds of many Western readers, "Yogi Breathing" suggests nothing more than a picture of a Hindu, sitting erect, and alternating nostrils in the act of breathing. "Only this and nothing more." We trust that this little work will open the eyes of the Western world to the great possibilities of Yogi Breathing, and the numerous methods whereby it may be employed.

THE GRAND YOGI PSYCHIC BREATH

The Yogis have a favorite form of psychic breathing which they practice occasionally, to which has been given a Sanskrit term of which the above is a general equivalent. We have given it last, as it requires practice on the part of the student in the line of rhythmic breathing and mental imagery, which he has now acquired by means of the preceding exercises. The general principles of the Grand Breath may be summed up in the old Hindu saying: "Blessed is the Yogi who can breathe through his bones." This exercise will fill the entire system with prana, and the student will emerge from it with every bone, muscle, nerve, cell, tissue, organ and part energized and attuned by the prana and the rhythm of the breath. It is a general housecleaning of the system, and he who practices it carefully will feel as if he had been given a new body, freshly created, from the crown of his head to the tips of his toes. We will let the exercise speak for itself.

1. Lie in a relaxed position, at perfect ease.
2. Breathe rhythmically until the rhythm is perfectly established.
3. Then, inhaling and exhaling, form the mental image of the breath being drawn up through the bones of the legs, and then forced out through them; then through the bones of the arms; then through the top of the skull; then through the stomach; then through the reproductive region; then as if it were traveling upward and downward along the spinal column; and then as if the breath were being inhaled and exhaled through every pore of the skin, the whole body being filled with prana and life.

4. Then (breathing rhythmically) send the current of prana to the Seven Vital Centers, in turn, as follows, using the mental picture as in previous exercises:
    (a) To the forehead.
    (b) To the back of the head.
    (c) To the base of the brain.
    (d) To the Solar Plexus.
    (e) To the Sacral Region (lower part of the spine).
    (f) To the region of the navel.
    (g) To the reproductive region.
5. Finish by sweeping the current of prana, to and fro from head to feet several times.
6. Finish with Cleansing Breath.

CHAPTER 16 - YOGI SPIRITUAL BREATHING

The Yogis not only bring about desired mental qualities and properties by will-power coupled with rhythmic breathing, but they also develop spiritual faculties, or rather aid in their unfoldment, in the same way. The Oriental philosophies teach that man has many faculties which are at present in a dormant state, but which will become unfolded as the race progresses. They also teach that man, by the proper effort of the will, aided by favorable conditions, may aid in the unfoldment of these spiritual faculties, and develop them much sooner than in the ordinary process of evolution. In other words, one may even now develop spiritual powers of consciousness which will not become the common property of the race until after long ages of gradual development under the law of evolution. In all of the exercises directed toward this end, rhythmic breathing plays an important part.

There is of course no mystic property in the breath itself which produces such wonderful results, but the rhythm produced by the Yogi breath is such as to bring the whole system, including the brain, under perfect control, and in perfect harmony, and by this means, the most perfect condition is obtained for the unfoldment of these latent faculties.

In this work we cannot go deeply into the philosophy of the East regarding spiritual development, because this subject would require volumes to cover it, and then again, the subject is too abstruse to interest the average reader. There are also other reasons, well known to occultists, why this knowledge should not be spread broadcast at this time.

Rest assured, dear student, that when the time comes for you to take the next step, the way will be opened out before you. "When the chela (student) is ready, the guru (master) appears." In this chapter we will give you directions for the development of two phases of spiritual consciousness, i.e., (1) the consciousness of the identity of the Soul, and (2) the consciousness of the connection of the Soul with the Universal Life. Both of the exercises given below are simple, and consist of mental images firmly held, accompanied with rhythmic breathing. The student must not expect too much at the start, but must make haste slowly, and be content to develop as does the flower, from seed to blossom.

SOUL CONSCIOUSNESS

The real Self is not the body or even the mind of man. These things are but a part of his personality, the lesser self. The real Self is the Ego, whose manifestation is in individuality. The real Self is independent of the body, which it inhabits, and is even independent of the mechanism of the mind, which it uses as an instrument. The real Self is a drop from the Divine Ocean, and is eternal and indestructible. It cannot die or be annihilated, and no matter what becomes of the body, the real Self still exists. It is the Soul. Do not think of your Soul as a thing apart from you, for YOU are the Soul, and the body is the unreal and transitory part of you which is changing in material every day, and which you will someday discard. You may develop the faculties so that they will be conscious of the reality of the Soul, and its independence of the body. The Yogi plan for such development is by meditation upon the real Self or Soul, accompanied by rhythmic breathing. The following exercise is the simplest form.

EXERCISE - Place your body in a relaxed, reclining position. Breathe rhythmically, and meditate upon the real Self, thinking of yourself as an entity independent of the body, although inhabiting it and being able to leave it at will. Think of yourself, not as the body, but as a spirit, and of your body as but a shell, useful and comfortable, but not a part of the real You. Think of yourself as an independent being, using the body only as a convenience. While meditating, ignore the body entirely, and you will find that you will often become almost entirely unconscious of it, and will seem to be out of the body to which you may return when you are through with the exercise.

This is the gist of the Yogi meditative breathing methods, and if persisted in will give one a wonderful sense of the reality of the Soul, and will make him seem almost independent of the body. The sense of immortality will often come with this increased consciousness, and the person will begin to show signs of spiritual development which will be noticeable to himself and others. But he must not allow himself to live too much in the upper regions, or to despise his body, for he is here on this plane for a purpose, and he must not neglect his opportunity to gain the experiences necessary to round him out, nor must he fail to respect his body, which is the Temple of the Spirit.

THE UNIVERSAL CONSCIOUSNESS

The Spirit in man, which is the highest manifestation of his Soul, is a drop in the ocean of Spirit, apparently separate and distinct, but yet really in touch with the ocean itself, and with every other drop in it. As man unfolds in spiritual consciousness, he becomes more and more aware of his relation to the Universal Spirit, or Universal Mind as some term it. He feels at times as if he were almost at-one-ment with it, and then again, he loses the sense of contact and relationship. The Yogis seek to attain this state of Universal Consciousness by meditation and rhythmic breathing, and many have thus attained the highest degree of spiritual attainment possible to man in this stage of his existence. The student of this work will not need the higher instruction regarding adeptship at this time, as he has much to do and accomplish before he reaches that stage, but it may be well to initiate him into the elementary stages of the Yogi exercises for developing Universal Consciousness, and if he is in earnest he will discover means and methods whereby he may progress. The way is always opened to him who is ready to tread the path. The following exercise will be found to do much toward developing the Universal Consciousness in those who faithfully practice it.

EXERCISE - Place your body in a reclining, relaxed position. Breathe rhythmically, and meditate upon your relationship with the Universal Mind of which you are but an atom. Think of yourself as being in touch with All, and at-one-ment with All. See All as One, and your Soul as a part of that One. Feel that you are receiving the vibrations from the great Universal Mind, and are partaking of its power and strength and wisdom. The two following lines of meditation may be followed.

(a) With each inhalation, think of yourself as drawing in to yourself the strength and power of the Universal Mind. When exhaling think of yourself as passing out to others that same power, at the same time being filled with love for every living thing, and desiring that it be a partaker of the same blessings which you are now receiving. Let the Universal Power circulate through you.

(b) Place your mind in a reverential state, and meditate upon the grandeur of the Universal Mind, and open yourself to the inflow of the Divine Wisdom, which will fill you with illuminating wisdom, and then let the same flow out from you to your brothers and sisters whom you love and would help.

This exercise leaves with those who have practiced it a new-found sense of strength, power and wisdom, and a feeling of spiritual exaltation and bliss. It must be practiced only in a serious, reverential mood, and must not be approached triflingly or lightly.

GENERAL DIRECTIONS

The exercises given in this chapter require the proper mental attitude and conditions, and the trifler and person of a non-serious nature, or one without a sense of spirituality and reverence, had better pass them by, as no results will be obtained by such persons, and besides it is a willful trifling with things of a high order, which course never benefits those who pursue it. These exercises are for the few who can understand them, and the others will feel no attraction to try them.

During meditation let the mind dwell upon the ideas given in the exercise, until it becomes clear to the mind, and gradually manifests in real consciousness within you. The mind will gradually become passive and at rest, and the mental image will manifest clearly. Do not indulge in these exercises too often, and do not allow the blissful state produced to render you dissatisfied with the affairs of everyday life, as the latter are useful and necessary for you, and you must never shirk a lesson, however disagreeable to you it may be. Let the joy arising from the unfolding consciousness buoy you up and nerve you for the trials of life, and not make you dissatisfied and disgusted. All is good, and everything has its place. Many of the students who practice these exercises will in time wish to know more. Rest assured that when the time comes, we will see that you do not seek in vain. Go on in courage and confidence, keeping your face toward the East, from whence comes the rising Sun.

Peace be unto you, and unto all men.

Printed in Great Britain
by Amazon